GASTROESOPHAGEAL CARCINOMA

CONTEMPORARY SURGICAL MANAGEMENT SERIES

- Joseph A. Caprini, M.D., John P. Fotopoulos, M.D., Miguel A. Oviedo, M.D., and Daniel Paloyan, M.D.: *Gallstones*
- Siroos S. Shirazi, M.D.: *Hernias of the Diaphragm and Abdominal Wall*
- James T. Anderson, M.D., Nathan W. Pearlman, M.D., and David N. Campbell, M.D.: *Gastroesophageal Carcinoma*

Books in Preparation:

- Robert H. Quinn, M.D., John B. Gregg, M.D., and C. Douglas Wood, M.D.: *Benign Diseases of the Esophagus*
- Lewis M. Flint, Jr., M.D. and Donald E. Fry, M.D. (eds.): *Surgical Infections*

CONTEMPORARY SURGICAL
MANAGEMENT SERIES

GASTROESOPHAGEAL CARCINOMA

James T. Anderson, M.D.
Associate Professor of Surgery
University of Colorado Health Sciences Center
Chief of Cardiothoracic Surgery
Denver Veterans Administration Hospital

Nathan W. Pearlman, M.D.
Assistant Professor of Surgery
University of Colorado Health Sciences Center
Chief of Oncology and Oncological Surgery
Denver Veterans Administration Hospital

David N. Campbell, M.D.
Assistant Professor of Surgery
University of Colorado Health Sciences Center
Denver Veterans Administration Hospital

Medical Examination Publishing Co., Inc.
an Excerpta Medica company

Anderson, James T.
Gastroesophageal carcinoma.

Bibliography: p.
Includes index.
1. Esophagogastric junction—Cancer—Surgery.
2. Esophagogastric junction—Cancer. I. Pearlman, Nathan W. II. Campbell, David N. III. Title.
(DNLM: 1. Esophageal neoplasms. 2. Stomach neoplasms.
3. Esophagogastric junction. WI 250 A547g)
RD668.3.A5 616.99'432 81-16778
ISBN 0-87488-829-8 AACR2

MEDICAL EXAMINATION PUBLISHING CO., INC.
an Excerpta Medica company
969 Stewart Avenue
Garden City, New York

January 1982

Printed in the United States of America

To the general and thoracic surgery residents of the University of Colorado Health Science Center and the Denver Veterans Administration Hospital who have provided a constant stimulus to analyze and refine the details of management necessary for a successful, aggressive approach to these difficult patient care problems.

Contents

	Preface	ix
1	Introduction, Epidemiology, and Etiology	1
2	Natural History and Prognosis	8
3	Clinical Manifestations and Diagnosis	14
4	Treatment of Gastroesophageal Carcinoma	39
5	Summary and Prognosis	114
	References	116
	Index	136

Preface

In this present treatise we have concentrated our discussion on carcinomas of the gastroesophageal junction which present clinically as management problems with certain characteristics distinct from those of carcinoma of the remainder of the esophagus or stomach. The pattern of lymphatic metastases, the surgical approach, the relative ineffectiveness of radiation therapy, and the etiological factors peculiar to carcinomas at this location justify such a specific discussion.

We have placed particular emphasis on the environmental factors contributing to the etiology of gastroesophageal carcinoma, the natural history and prognosis of carcinomas of the gastroesophageal junction, the clinical manifestations of tumors of this location and the steps in diagnosis, the role of various forms of therapy for these tumors with particular emphasis on a scheme of selective therapy based on the stage of the carcinoma and the general condition of the patient, and finally (but possibly most importantly), a detailed discussion of the fine points in preoperative, operative, and postoperative care of patients undergoing surgical resection for cure or palliation.

Our hope is that this book will aid both the beginning and the experienced esophageal surgeon in refining his selection of therapy for gastroesophageal carcinomas and his surgical care.

We would like to express particular gratitude to Mr. R.J. M. McCormack and Mr. Philip Walbaum of Edinburgh, and Dr. R. K. Brown of Denver, Colorado, who were our mentors in esophageal surgery and to Ms. Teresa Carlson for her efforts in the preparation of the manuscript.

notice

Chapter 1

INTRODUCTION, EPIDEMIOLOGY, AND ETIOLOGY

The term gastroesophageal cancer is often used for squamous or adenocarcinomas found at the gastroesophageal junction. Although many authors group these lesions with those arising more proximal in the esophagus, they are not distinct pathologic entities but rather a mixture of proximal gastric and distal esophageal tumors. One might easily wonder, therefore, as to the merits of discussing gastroesophageal neoplasms as if they were a distinct entity. There are several reasons for doing so. First, there continues to be much disagreement over how to best manage cancers of the cervical or upper two-thirds of the esophagus, whereas this is not the case for distal third lesions and most authorities would agree that the latter are best treated surgically whenever possible. Second, the epidemiology and natural history of adenocarcinoma of the gastroesophageal junction is very similar to squamous carcinoma of the esophagus, more so, in fact, than to adenocarcinomas of the body or antrum of the stomach. Third, the treatment of gastroesophageal tumors, whether by surgery, radiation, or other measures, tends to be the same in most instances, regardless of histology. Finally, although many decry its use, the term gastroesophageal cancer continues to be used directly or indirectly in the literature, suggesting that it is a separate clinical entity in the minds of many authors.

About 11 to 16% of gastric cancers involve the gastroesophageal junction, as do 30 to 50% of those originating in the esophagus (1-10). As a result, the histology of these lesions is adenocarcinoma in 60 to 70% of patients and squamous cancer in the other 30 to 40% (1-10). Since primary adenocarcinoma of the esophagus comprises only 1 to 2% of all malignancies in that organ (11, 12), one can assume that virtually all adenocarcinomas found at the gastroesophageal junction arose from gastric mucosa. One can also presume that virtually all squamous cancers of this region came from the esophagus, because primary squamous cancer of the stomach is rare and has only been described in or around the pylorus (13). Cell types other than squamous or adenocarcinoma are unlikely to be encountered in this region. Lymphosarcoma, oat cell carcinoma, carcinosarcoma, rhabdomyosarcoma, adenoid cystic carcinoma, and mucoepidermoid carcinoma of the esophagus have all been described (14-20), but are rare enough as to seem to warrant a case report each time one is found. Primary lymphomas and leiomyosarcomas of the stomach are not that rare; however, the former makes up only about 1% of gastric malignancies and the latter, a smaller fraction (13). In addition, each of these gastric tumors tends to occur in portions of the stomach which are distal to the cardia.

The incidence of gastroesophageal cancer cannot be determined with accuracy because, as mentioned earlier, some authors consider these lesions to be esophageal tumors while others group them with gastric cancer. In spite of that, some estimates as to their frequency can be made. Current projections for the number of new gastric cancers to be diagnosed in the United States in 1980 are 23,000 cases, while the estimated number of new esophageal cancers is 8800 (21). If, as suggested earlier, the gastroesophageal junction is involved in 11 to 16% of the former cases, and 30 to 50% of the latter, the number of gastroesophageal tumors will be somewhere in the range of 5000 to 8000 cases.

The epidemiology of these malignancies is not a separate subject, but rather a combination of the epidemiologic factors relating to gastric and esophageal cancer. Both malignancies demonstrate rather marked geographic variations in frequency and this is probably also true for tumors of the gastroesophageal region. For instance, incidence rates for gastric cancer in men range from 70 to 95 cases per 100,000 in Iceland, Chile, or Japan, to 20 to 25 per 100,000 in Great Britain, Sweden, or Canada (22,23). Incidence rates among men in the United States are even lower, 13.7 cases per 100,000 (22,23). The frequency of gastric cancer in women in these countries, as well as in most others, is one-half to two-thirds of that found in men. As a result, the male/female ratio for this disease remains fairly constant at 2:1 or 3:2 in most parts of the world (23).

Esophageal cancer not only varies markedly in frequency between different countries, but between different regions of the same country as well. China has 135 cases per 100,000 in some provinces but only 1.4 per 100,000 in others (24). Incidence rates in the Caspian Littoral of Iran range from 70 per 100,000 in the eastern part of the region to 6 per 100,000 in the west, a distance of approximately 800 miles (25,26). Males living in the Transkei or Natal region of South Africa have 70.4 and 40.9 cases per 100,000 respectively, as compared to 5.8 per 100,000 among Cape Province "colored" males and 2.4 per 100,000 among Ibadan males in Nigeria (27,28). Black males in the United States demonstrate the same phenomenon. While cancer of the esophagus is three times more frequent among this cohort than among white males (15.6 versus 5 cases per 100,000), this is not a uniform finding throughout the country (29). Thus, black males in Birmingham, Alabama, are found to have incidence rates nearly as low as those in white (7.4 per 100,000), while the rates for black males in Pittsburgh or Atlanta are 20 per 100,000 (28). Finally, it would appear that the incidence of esophageal cancer is higher in France than in any other European country (13.6 cases per 100,000); yet most of the cases accrue from three western provinces and much fewer from the south of the country (29).

The male/female ratio for esophageal cancer also varies with location, in contrast to that for gastric cancer. In Iran, this figure is almost 1:1, whereas it is 4:1 in the United States, 9:1 in South Africa, and almost 13:1 in France (27-30). Adenocarcinoma of the cardia is like squamous cancer of the esophagus in this regard, for its male/female ratio ranges from 4:1 to 7:1 (31,32).

The age range for these two malignancies is 20 to 90 years; however, most patients are between 50 and 70 years of age. The predilection for development of gastric cancer, on the other hand, appears to be acquired early in life because as groups migrate from high- to low-incidence regions, their frequency of disease only begins to drop with succeeding generations (23,33). This may also occur with esophageal cancer but, as yet, has not been investigated in depth.

Another interesting feature of the epidemiology of gastric cancer is its decline in frequency over the past three to four decades. This has occurred among all races and sexes in western Europe and North America (23) and now appears to have occurred more recently in Japan, as well (34). In contrast, the incidence of esophageal cancer during this period has either remained stable or actually increased (21,27,28,35).

Major risk factors for esophageal cancer in most parts of the world appear to be alcohol, tobacco, and low socioeconomic class (27,28,35-38). The one region where this does not appear to be the case is the Caspian Littoral of Iran, where the Moslem population neither smokes nor drinks to any extent, if at all (26). Major risk factors in this region seem to be diets consisting mainly of bread, sheep and goat's milk, as well as deficiencies in riboflavin, zinc, vitamin A, and vitamin C (26, 39).

Low socioeconomic class is a significant risk factor for cancer of the stomach as well, with incidence rates being 2.5 times higher in such groups (23). The roles played by alcohol and tobacco are less clear in this disease, however, than in esophageal cancer. Zacho et al (40), found the incidence of gastric cancer to be about the same in smokers and nonsmokers. Male smokers who did develop gastric cancer, however, tended to have more tumors of the cardia and less of the body or antrum, suggesting another similarity between malignancies of the cardia and those of the esophagus. Other authors have suggested a role for alcohol and tobacco in the epidemiology of cancer of the cardia (32,41), but their documentation was incomplete.

The other major environmental risk factors for cancer of the stomach are dietary. Some of the highest incidence rates in the world for this tumor occur in regions where diets contain large amounts of smoked food, salt-dried fish, and pickled vegetables (23,42). In the United States, the frequency of disease appears to correlate with diets rich in starch, but low in protein, fresh fruit, and fresh vegetables (43). Finally, living in regions where nitrates are used extensively for fertilizer and/or can be found in the local drinking water would also appear to add to the risk for this malignancy (42,44).

In addition to these exogenous risk factors, certain endogenous conditions have also been associated with each tumor. Pernicious anemia is felt by many to be a premalignant condition because it so often is followed by the development of gastric cancer (23). Blood group A is also often quoted as a risk factor for cancer of the stomach, but in fact the incidence among such groups is only 1.2 times greater than among other blood types (23). The role of reflux esophagitis may also be important. McDonald found that 35% of patients with cancer of the cardia had a hiatus hernia and 24% had a history of "heartburn," whereas this was true for only 6% of those with neoplasms of other regions of the stomach and 13% of patients with squamous cancer of the esophagus (32). Neaf et al., in a review of 6000 endoscopies (45), found that 1% of patients with reflux esophagitis had coexistent cancer of the gastroesophageal junction, an incidence of 1000 cases per 100,000.

There would also appear to be some deleterious factor contributed by previous gastric resection. Stalsberg and Taksdal (46) noted that, while the frequency of previous gastric surgery among patients with gastric cancer was no higher than in matched controls when such operations were performed 15 years ago or less, it was 6 times higher if operated on 25 years ago or more previously. Schrumpf and associates (47) reported finding a much higher incidence of early gastric cancer when routine endoscopy and multiple random biopsies of normal areas were carried out on patients 20 to 25 years after a partial gastrectomy. Nicholls found the incidence of gastric cancer to be 1.3% in patients who had undergone a partial gastrectomy for ulcers of the stomach, but only 0.01% in those who had such an operation for a duodenal ulcer (the latter incidence was no different from that seen in the general population) (48). Finally, MacGregor estimates that malignant change occurs in 10% of patients with atrophic gastritis (49), a condition very often seen following partial gastrectomy.

Endogenous conditions which may predispose to the development of esophageal cancer are achalasia, long-standing caustic strictures, and, perhaps, scleroderma. The incidence of cancer of the esophagus in patients with achalasia is variously quoted as being in the range of 0.6 to 8% (50-52). Postlethwait, however, in a large review of the literature found the figure to be closer to 2% (53) and this may be a better estimation of the risk. Patients with caustic strictures of the esophagus are also known to be at somewhat higher risk for malignant degeneration; however, the magnitude of this problem is not clear. Postlethwait found the incidence of previous caustic burns to be 1.4 to 1.6% in patients with known esophageal cancer, but the numbers of cancer in those with strictures remains a mystery. Finally, it would appear that scleroderma may also predispose to the development of esophageal cancer (54); however, the latter condition is rare and impinges negligibly on overall incidence rates.

As judged by the foregoing, the major etiologic factors in both gastric and esophageal cancer would appear to be environmental in most parts of the world. It is not clear at this time, however, exactly what agents are present in the environment of high-risk groups so as to predispose them to the development of each tumor. Many investigators feel that the best candidates for such a role are the family of nitrosamines and nitrosamides. These chemicals are potent carcinogens in laboratory animals and have induced both esophageal and gastric cancer in a variety of species (55-60). In most instances, the method used for such purposes has been to add small amounts of one of these agents to the animals' drinking water, a method by which humans might also be exposed to such chemicals. The esophageal tumors induced in these animals are uniformly squamous cancers, while the gastric lesions are adenocarcinomas. On occasion, both cell types will be found in the same animal (59). One study also suggests that the carcinogenic influence of nitrosamines is greater in the young and males of a species than in adults or females, observations which also seem to mirror epidemiologic findings in humans (60).

Although nitrosamines or nitrosamides may not be major carcinogenic influences in humans, which remains to be seen, there are certainly a large number of sources in the environment for exposure to such agents. Tobacco smoke, a risk factor for at least esophageal cancer, has been found to contain several nonvolatile nitrosamines which can be used to induce tumors of the esophagus in rats, mice, and Syrian hamsters (61). Some varieties of beer have also been found to contain trace amounts of these chemicals (62). Wine may have the capacity to catalyze the formation of nitrosamines in vitro (63). The capacity might be potentially retained when the wine is ingested. Chronic use of alcohol also tends to be followed by serum and tissue deficiencies in riboflavin, zinc, and vitamin A (64). Such deficiencies have been used to promote the carcinogenicity of various chemicals in animals (64) and have been correlated with the incidence of esophageal cancer in humans (26,39).

Foods grown in certain parts of the world constitute another potential source of nitrosamines. The soil in regions of China where esophageal cancer is endemic, as well as in the Transkei, appears to be deficient in molybdenum, and nitrosamines have been found in food grown in both regions (24,65). A postulated explanation for this association is that plants absorb most of their nitrogen in the form of nitrate and need molybdenum to reduce it to ammonia (65). Molybdenum deficiency could, therefore, lead to nitrate buildup in the plant and be followed by spontaneous formation of nitrous acid. The latter would tend to react with secondary amines already present in most plants and produce nitrosamines. Whether this proposed scenario actually takes place is unproven, but the fact that nitrosamines do occur in food grown in molybdenum deficient soil is intriguing.

A third source of these chemicals is endogenous production in the stomach. Mirvish has demonstrated that citrulline, arginine, and methylguanidine will react with nitrites and form nitrosamines when acid conditions similar to those found in the human stomach are present (66). He has also shown that this reaction is blocked by ascorbic acid (67), a vitamin conspicuously lacking in the diet of groups at high risk for esophageal and gastric cancer. Endo and Takahashi noted that the nitrosated methylguanidine formed in gastric juice was mutagenic in bacterial cultures at a 16-fold dilution (68). Hill et al. (43) have presented evidence that bacteria will catalyze the nitrosation of amines in the absence of an acid milieu. Bayland and Walker (69) report that thiocyanate, which is found in human saliva and gastric juice, can also act as a catalyst for this process.

It would appear, therefore, that conditions which increase levels of nitrate, nitrite, or secondary amines in the stomach, as well as those which add bacteria or thiocyanate to this milieu, are potentially more carcinogenic than those which do not. In this light, it would seem of interest that Raineri and Weisburger have found that boiled potatoes and a commonly used stew preparation develop significant amounts of endogenous nitrite when left at room temperature overnight, whereas this did not occur when the food was kept refrigerated (70). Food items such as boiled potatoes and stew are commonly in frequent use by low socioeconomic groups, and the refrigeration facilities for storage of such items between meals may not always be ideal. As such, these groups may be ingesting more preformed nitrites than desirable. Salt-dried fish, another risk factor for gastric cancer, has been found to contain large amounts of secondary amines, whereas this was not the case for fresh fish, beef, and chicken (71). In some instances, salt-dried fish has also been found to contain nitrosamines (72). Salted vegetables in soy sauce, another food item favored by groups at high risk for cancer of the stomach, led to markedly increased mitotic counts of gastric mucosa when fed to volunteers in one study (73). Thiocyanate concentrations have been found to be two to four times higher in the gastric juice and saliva of smokers than in nonsmokers (68, 74). Finally, Ruddell et al. (74) noted that nitrite levels in gastric juice of patients with duodenal ulcers or normal stomachs are around 1.7 umol/liter, whereas they are 25 to 38 umol/liter in the gastric juice of patients with achlorhydria or proven cancer of the stomach.

Thus, there is a large body of evidence implicating the nitrosamines and nitrosamides in the etiology of human gastric and esophageal cancer. More work needs to be done in this area before the relationship can be solidified. Until that time, the association between these chemicals and human malignancy will remain tantalizing but, unfortunately, speculative.

Chapter 2

NATURAL HISTORY AND PROGNOSIS

The natural history of gastroesophageal cancer is characterized in most patients by a progressive compromise in the lumen of the distal esophagus and then a spread to other sites. At least 90% of patients complain of dysphagia when they present with an average weight loss of 20 to 30 lbs (4, 75). Appelqvist (75) found that 10 to 20% of patients were so debilitated at the time of diagnosis that only palliative measures could be contemplated. Another 10 to 30% were inoperable on the basis of obvious local spread of disease or distant metastases. Other authors have not addressed the reasons for inoperability in such detail; however, the findings in the studies of Gunnlaugsson et al. (2) and Stone et al. (4) that show 40 to 50% of patients either never coming to surgery or undergoing only a laparotomy mirror the number of inoperable cases in Appelqvist's experience.

The fact that about half the patients with this disease are inoperable when they present is often ascribed to a lack of serosal covering for the esophagus, which allows it to dilate for long periods of time, and often to considerable size, without causing symptoms. Skinner has estimated, in fact, that at least 90% of the circumference of this organ must be involved with tumor before dysphagia ensues (6). While this is undoubtedly part of the explanation for delays in diagnosis, it would appear that patient delay in seeking medical attention also contributes. The average duration of dysphagia which is admitted, is four to six months in most series (4, 75). Our conversations with family members, however, suggest that many of these patients were aware of swallowing difficulties much earlier than this, but chose not to do anything about them. Exact reasons for this are always unclear, but alcohol may play a role. It is a major dietary item for many of these patients and, being a liquid, is often the last to be obstructed by the tumor. Its analgesic effects may also allow the patient to gain relief of minor to moderate degrees of pain, symptoms which would otherwise propel him/her to the doctor at an earlier time. Whatever the actual reasons, it is unfortunate that so many of these patients currently are diagnosed at a time when only palliation can be offered.

Other major local signs and symptoms of the tumor are substernal or epigastric pain, bleeding, and cough. Pain is mentioned by 20 to 50% of patients (4, 75) and may be intermittent or constant. In most instances the pain associated with this disease is burning in nature and situated anteriorly. Some patients, however, complain of a pain which is dull, constant, and which radiates through to the back. This is an ominous sign, for it generally connotes a lesion which has invaded the retroperitoneum or posterior mediastinum. While cancers of this sort can occasionally be resected to restore swallowing, they are unlikely to be amenable to complete resection in hopes of a cure.

Bleeding occurs in about 7 to 20% of cases (4, 75) and is usually a slow blood loss, causing melena and/or minor degrees of hematemesis. Such bleeding is usually due to superficial slough of the tumor and does not tend to be massive on any given occasion, although it can lead to rather significant anemia. Cancers of the esophagus can on occasion erode into the aorta and this potentially could occur with those of the gastroesophageal junction. While this has generally occurred following radiotherapy (76), it has also been reported in the absence of such treatment (77). Thus, if a patient with a gastroesophageal tumor shows evidence of massive hemorrhage into the gut, the possibility of an aortoesophageal fistula should be kept in mind.

Cough of a significant nature is complained of by about 5 to 10% of patients (4, 75) and is usually due to persistent aspiration of food or saliva, which is retained in the esophagus when the patient is supine or asleep. This can lead to a significant loss of pulmonary reserve and/or a pneumonia which persists despite appropriate antibiotics and tracheobronchial toilet.

Local spread of these tumors tends to be both extramural and intramural. The incidence of extraesophageal disease ranges from 16% in the series of Gunnlaugsson et al. (2), to 30 to 40% in the studies of Magill and Stevenson (1), Skinner (6), and Appelqvist (75). Appelqvist suggests that the presence of extraesophageal cancer may be predicted by the size of the tumor. Thus, he found that lesions 4 cm or less in length had extramural extension in 8% of instances, whereas such disease occurred in 24% of tumors 4 to 8 cm long and 34% of those over 8 cm (75). With early stages of extraesophageal spread, only those lymph nodes and/or portions of the diaphragm which are immediately adjacent to the distal esophagus may be invaded, and these can usually be resected in continuity with the tumor without undue morbidity or mortality. Unfortunately, this extent of spread is not usually encountered, and one more frequently finds that the tumor has invaded the celiac axis, retroperitoneum, body and/or tail of the pancreas, left lobe of the liver, or hilum of the spleen. This involvement generally precludes resection for cure.

Intramural, or submucosal, invasion is another common route for these cancers to spread and it may go on for rather significant distance without being apparent grossly. While this fact would appear to be rather well-known, the literature fails to give a clear idea of the extent of submucosal invasion likely to be encountered clinically. In the studies of Burgess et al. (5) and Appelqvist (75), 80 to 90% of the submucosal invasion seen was confined to within 2 cm of the gross limits of the tumor. These measurements, however, were made on specimens which had been removed and fixed in formalin. The shrinkage seen in these circumstances could easily underestimate the amount of spread which is encountered clinically. That this may be the case is suggested to by the studies of Scanlon et al. (78), and Sefton et al (3). In the former work, it was found that 45. 6% of patients undergoing a segmental esophagectomy for cancer either developed suture line recurrences or had positive resection margins when the surgeon felt that such margins were "adequate." Presumably, this would mean greater than 2 cm. In the latter study, 55% of patients had positive resection margins during esophagogastrectomy when such margins were 6 cm wide. Even more surprising was Sefton's finding that positive resection margins occurred more often with adenocarcinoma than with squamous cancer. In our experience, a margin of 6 or 7 cm is usually taken on either side of the tumor and generally is free of tumor. These margins are always checked with frozen section, however, and occasionally the finding of submucosal tumor has necessitated extending the resection much further than planned, usually in a proximal direction.

The lymphatic spread of gastroesophageal tumors tends to be the same, regardless of their histology. The first echelon of nodes likely to be involved lie adjacent to the distal esophagus, along the proximal lesser curve of the stomach and along the route of the left gastric artery. Further spread then tends to be found in the celiac axis nodes, those on the dorsum of the pancreas or in the hilum of the spleen, near the left adrenal gland and along the hepatic artery (79-81). The incidence of nodal metastasis at surgery is about 50% for squamous cancers and 60 to 70% for adenocarcinomas (1,2,4,82,83).

Distant metastases tend to be most frequently found in the liver, lungs, or peritoneal surfaces beyond the gastroesophageal junction. About 16% of patients also have metastases to the adrenal glands at autopsy, most often occurring in the context of widespread disease elsewhere (84). Appelqvist found that 6% of patients also had spread to supraclavicular nodes at autopsy (75). Bone metastases occur in about 5% of patients with squamous cancer of the esophagus (85); however, the incidence is lower in those with adenocarcinomas of the cardia. Hypercalcemia is commonly encountered in widespread squamous cancer of the esophagus and might be interpreted to mean that bone metastases are present. This does not appear to be the case in most patients, however, for both Stephens et al. (86) and Chandrasekhara et al. (87) were unable to document such bone involvement in more than two-thirds of the cases they reviewed.

The incidence of distant metastases, when the patient presents, is difficult to determine with accuracy, because patients are often considered too incurable because of advanced local disease as well as from distant spread. Thus, 40 to 50% of patients in the studies of Gunnlaugsson et al. (2) and Appelqvist (75) do not undergo resections; however, the reasons for this include poor physical condition, advanced regional disease, as well as distant metastases. Magill and Simmons found previously occult spread to the liver or peritoneum in 13% of patients at laparotomy; however, the number with distant disease which was diagnosed preoperatively is not given (1). In the study of Van Andel and associates (7), there are 328 patients with squamous carcinoma of the esophagus, of whom only 67 (20%) were considered incurable at the outset. Another 115 patients (35%) were felt to be inoperable because of local spread of disease and received curative attempts at radiation. The fact that only 20% of the latter group lived a year suggests that the incidence of distant metastases was much higher than suspected prior to instituting radiotherapy. Finally, in the study of Ellis and Gibb (88), there are 153 potential candidates for esophagogastrectomy with 124 (81%) coming to operation and 102 (67%) undergoing resection. About one-fourth of these were palliative resections, however, suggesting that only half the patients had disease confined to the immediate region of the gastroesophageal junction.

The prognosis for patients with gastroesophageal cancer is a function of the stage of disease present at diagnosis, histology of the tumor, and how it is treated. There is not presently available a staging system for only lesions of the gastroesophageal junction. One does exist for tumors of the esophagus, however, and does seem relatively applicable to gastroesophageal neoplasms (89). In this system, the disease is characterized as in Table 1.

It is apparent that this staging system is fairly inaccurate in the absence of laparotomy, particularly in terms of being able to determine the extent of intraabdominal disease. It would be useful, however, to try and fit gastroesophageal into these categories, because that is the only means by which treatment results can be compared between various centers, and the influence of various treatment modalities on survival can be accurately determined. We have, therefore, attempted to review the published studies within the context of the TNM system, in hopes of providing some insight as to how stage determines prognosis.

Table 1 TMN Staging System for Carcinoma of the Esophagus

Primary Tumor (T):

TO	No demonstrable tumor in the esophagus
T1S	Carcinoma in situ
T1	A tumor less than 5 cm in length, with no obstruction radiographically or circumferential involvement, and without extraesophageal spread
T2	A tumor more than 5 cm without extraesophageal spread; or of any length and associated with obstruction or circumferential involvement; but without extraesophageal spread
T3	Any lesion which has evidence of extraesophageal spread

Node Involvement (N):

NX	Not assessed (clinical evaluation)
NO	Negative nodes (surgical evaluation)
N1	Positive nodes (surgical evaluation)

Distant Metastases (M):

MX	Not assessed
MO	No (known) distant metastases
M1	Distant metastases present

Stage Grouping:

Stage I:	T1 NO MO; or T1 NX MO
Stage II:	T2 NO MO; or T2 NX MO
Stage III:	Any T3; or any N1; or any M1

To facilitate this, tumors described by the subjective appelation resectable for cure will be considered T1 or T2 lesions, while those which are removed for palliation will be considered T3. Patients with positive nodes (N1) as well as those who do undergo a palliative resection will be placed in the resectable stage III category. Those who are considered inoperable or who undergo anything less than a resection (laparotomy, palliative intubation) will be considered to have unresectable stage III disease. When viewed in this context, one finds that esophagogastrectomy for stage I or II disease is associated with an average survival of 24 to 40 months and a five-year salvage of 20 to 35% (1, 2, 4, 83, 91). The same procedure in resectable stage III disease carries with it an average survival of 6 to 18 months and a 0 to 15% chance of living five years (1,2,4,82,83,91). While less than ideal, this is still better than the prognosis for patients with unresectable stage III lesions. Although palliative radiation, intubation, or both modalities in combination will allow about 50% of such patients to swallow reasonably well (92-95), average survival in this situation is only 2 to 5 months and few, if any, of these individuals live out the year (1,2,7,91-95).

The influence of tumor histology on prognosis is somewhat easier to quantify. In most studies, patients with squamous cancer are found to do better, stage for stage, than those with adenocarcinoma. Five-year survival for the former cell type in the series of Gunnlaugsson et al. (2) is 50% when nodes are negative and 15 to 20% when they are positive. Corresponding figures for adenocarcinomas are 27% to 7.6% survival, according to nodal status. Squamous cancers treated by esophagogastrectomy in the studies of Hankins et al. (82,90) were associated with a 26-month average survival and 21% five-year salvage as compared to six month average survival for adenocarcinoma, with no patient in the latter group living longer than 18 months. Not all authors find this prognostic difference by histology, however, and the five-year survival in the series of Magill and Simmons is about the same for both squamous and adenocarcinoma, 8% and 9%.

Treatment is also a major factor in prognosis but is exceedingly difficult to clarify. The major reason for this is that patients with the smaller tumors and a better prognosis thereto tend to be those operated on, while those with the larger lesions and/or distant metastases tend to be sent to the radiotherapist or managed with intubation. Because of this, one cannot determine how patients with a given stage of disease would do if treated by alternate methods. This does not constitute a call for trying alternate methods of treatment in stage I or II disease, but rather an acknowledgment of the fact that the influence of therapy on survival, in these stages, is exceedingly difficult if not impossible to quantify.

Chapter 3

CLINICAL MANIFESTATIONS AND DIAGNOSIS

Carcinoma of the esophagus is an insidious lesion with no early symptoms or signs that signal the presence of the disease, and cure is often not possible because metastatic disease is present or local invasion of vital structures has occurred by the time symptoms cause the patient to seek medical attention. The late presentation of symptoms is integrally related to the anatomic position of the esophagus and gastric cardia deep in the chest and the unique absence of serosa around the esophagus. With no investing serosa the esophagus can be distended asymptomatically to a much greater degree than other areas of the gastrointestinal tract; therefore, any lesion in the esophagus which causes only partial obstruction will usually be asymptomatic.

SYMPTOMS

Carcinoma of the gastroesophageal junction often does not cause clinical symptoms until over 90% of the lumen is involved with tumor (6). As the tumor grows the remaining wall of the esophagus dilates to maintain the lumen (Fig. 1), so that the tumor may be quite large before the lumen is narrowed. When the lumen is critically narrowed, dysphagia is experienced by the patient. Dysphagia is the sensation of difficulty swallowing or the sensation of food sticking in the esophagus; it is the most common initial presentation of carcinoma of the esophagus at any level, occurring in over 50% of the patients. Initially the dysphagis occurs with solid foods only, but as the tumor grows and the esophagus becomes less distensible, liquids become difficult to pass as well. Carcinoma of the gastroesophageal junction may initially give the sensation of difficulty swallowing in the high esophagus, rather than the true area of obstruction in the distal esophagus. The reason for this is unknown. As the tumor grows the patient begins to localize the "food sticking" sensation to the true area of obstruction. Dysphagia is the major symptom which alarms the patient enough to make him seek medical attention; however, there is often a delay between the time the patient first notes the onset of dysphagia and the time he presents to the physician for diagnosis. The average time for this delay as shown by LeRoux (96) is four months. Often vague symptoms such as indigestion, fullness, or a feeling of pressure may be present well in advance of dysphagia, but are so nonspecific that they cause no alarm to the patient. The diagnosis of carcinoma should always be considered when an adult presents with acute foreign body obstruction (usually a large food bolus) in the esophagus.

Pain is an uncommon initial presentation for carcinoma of the gastroesophageal junction or anywhere else in the esophagus, and when it is present it usually implies spread of the cancer outside the wall of the esophagus. The nerve supply to the esophagus consists of sympathetic and parasympathetic nerves, and pain is poorly transmitted by these fibers but is well transmitted by pain fibers in the aortic adventitia or prevertebral fascia.

Aspiration pneumonitis with cough, fever, and productive sputum is common and results from the inability to swallow secretions secondary to almost total obstruction of the esophageal lumen. Hoarseness secondary to recurrent nerve invasion occurs in upper esophageal tumors, but less frequently in tumors located at the gastroesophageal junction. Gross hematemesis is rare and may imply involvement of the aorta. These patients survive only a short period of time, and expire from massive bleeding from the vascular enteric fistula. Finally, general inanition with weight loss and weakness is often present by the time the patient presents to the physician, simply because he has been unable to eat.

SIGNS

Because symptoms occur so late in the growth of gastroesophageal carcinoma, metastatic disease is present in over 50% of the patients at the time of initial presentation (97). This tumor spreads by three common means: (1) local invasion; (2) lymphatic spread; and (3) blood vessel invasion. Local invasion may involve the diaphragm, pericardium, heart, pulmonary structures, and aorta. Lymphatic spread occurs first in the submucosal lymphatics of the esophagus and the paraesophageal nodes. Afterward, downward spread occurs to the gastric, celiac axis, splenic and pancreatic nodes, followed by nodes in the porta hepatis and periaortic nodes. Spread may occur upward to the perihilar, subcarinal, peritracheal, and supraclavicular nodes.

Finally, blood vessel invasion is responsible for liver, lung, bone, kidney, and adrenal metastases. Carcinoma of the gastroesophageal junction rarely involves the trachea because the anatomic bifurcation of the trachea occurs well above the area of the tumor. Tracheoesophageal fistulae as occur with lesions of the high and midesophagus, therefore, rarely occur; bronchoscopy, which is mandatory in the preoperative evaluation of cancers of the high and midesophagus, is usually not necessary in the evaluation of carcinoma located at the esophagogastric junction.

Examination of the patient often reveals no significant physical findings except general inanition, but a complete examination is still important. Palpation of lymph nodes in the supraclavicular area of Virchow may reveal metastatic disease. Tumors of the mid and upper esophagus tend to metastasize to the right supraclavicular area, while tumors of the lower esophagus and esophagogastric junction tend to metastasize to the left supraclavicular area and may occur without involvement of the intervening mediastinal nodes by seeding through the thoracic duct. Examination of the abdomen may reveal an enlarged liver suggestive of metastatic disease. Tumor nodules in the liver may be palpable depending on the thinness of the patient's abdominal wall. An epigastric mass may be present and can represent a large tumor mass in the stomach or a large mass of tumor nodes, both are ominous. A rectal examination may reveal a Blummers Shelf from peritoneal seeding of the rectal shelf. Again, the main point to be stressed is that because of its location deep in the chest, carcinoma of the esophagus presents with no specific physical signs suggestive of the diagnosis, and the physical findings that may be present suggest metastatic and hence incurable disease.

LABORATORY STUDIES

Routine laboratory tests are not useful in the diagnosis of carcinoma of the gastroesophageal junction. However, they are useful in evaluating the general condition of the patient. Abnormalities should be corrected especially if the patient is an operative candidate. A complete blood count may reveal a microcytic anemia from chronic blood loss secondary to the tumor, or more uncommonly, may reveal a normocytic, normochromic anemia from bone marrow metastases of the carcinoma. A review of routine chemistries may reveal abnormal electrolytes or an elevated blood urea and creatinine on the basis of dehydration and muscle breakdown. Serum total protein and albumin will give a gross indication of nutrition. Baseline clotting studies, a prothrombin time, partial thromboplastin time, and platelet count, should be obtained. Abnormal prothrombin time may occur on the basis of decreased vitamin K intake, so it may be necessary to give intramuscular vitamin K to return the prothrombin time to normal. Liver function tests may indicate the possibility of metastatic disease particularly if the alkaline phosphatase is elevated. The alkaline phosphatase may also be elevated on the basis of bone metastases; therefore, specific enzyme fractionation and a serum gamma-glutamic transferase may be important to differentiate the organ which is primarily involved. It is important, however, to keep in mind that many patients with carcinoma of the esophagus also have intrinsic liver disease on the basis of alcoholic injury, since carcinoma of the esophagus is often closely associated with heavy alcoholic consumption. Alcoholic liver disease more often causes elevation of the serum glutamic-oxaloacetic transaminase and the serum glutamic-pyruvic transaminase.

A standard chest film (PA and lateral views) should be obtained and may show the presence of metastatic disease to the lungs (Fig. 2), the presence of aspiration pneumonitis, and/or some degree of chronic pulmonary disease. Most of the patients with carcinoma of esophagus have an associated heavy smoking history, and chronic obstructive pulmonary disease is common. Arterial blood gases and pulmonary function tests are of value to document this and to establish the severity of the disease.

RADIOLOGIC DIAGNOSIS

Dysphagia is not a sine qua non of carcinoma of the esophagus and occurs with other benign lesions of the esophagus such as reflux esophagitis with stricture, achalasia, and diffuse esophageal spasm. In fact, anything which disrupts motility will cause dysphagia, but in a patient over the age of 40, carcinoma must be the primary diagnosis until it is absolutely shown not to be present by a comprehensive evaluation. Following a thorough history and physical examination, a high index of suspicion should prompt the physician to obtain a barium esophagram and upper gastrointestinal series. Because of the variety of radiologic patterns, carcinoma of distal esophagus may be mimicked by other benign esophageal lesions. However, sufficient characteristic features of carcinoma of the esophagus such as rigidity, nodularity, of shelf-like margins will usually be present to make an accurate diagnosis. According to Bruni and Nelson, radiographic studies will be accurate in the diagnosis of carcinoma of the esophagus about 90% of the time (98). Wiot and Nelson state that there are three relatively distinct radiographic configurations of carcinoma of the esophagus: infiltrative, polypoid, and ulcerative (99). The infiltrative form is the most common type and spreads in the wall of the esophagus (Fig. 3), The proximal and distal margins of the infiltrative type are usually tapered, but an annular variant is sometimes seen. The lumen appears to be narrowed in a concentric manner. The second most common form is the polypoid lesion (Fig. 4). This generally appears as irregular polypoid filling defects, usually localized, but at times quite extensive. The third form is the ulcerative form, and this is relatively uncommon. The ulceration tends to occupy much of the length of the tumor. Carcinoma of the gastric cardia may present as a gastric mass with upward extension into the esophagus (Fig. 5). An important radiologic sign of carcinoma is the corner sign. This is a step-off, or indentation at one of the proximal margins, and though not infallible in the diagnosis of carcinoma, it is one of the best signs to distinguish carcinoma from benign disease (Fig. 6-8). The proximal esophagus will rarely be distended in carcinoma of the esophagus to the extent typical of achalasia since the obstruction is of shorter duration. Also, in achalasia the esophagus tapers down distally to a smooth neck (Fig. 9). Benign disease, such as intraluminal leiomyoma (Fig. 10) or Schatzki's Ring (Fig. 11), have a smooth mucosal outline on barium swallow, whereas malignant disease of the esophagus has a shaggy moth-eaten appearance to the mucosa (Fig. 12). Extrinsic masses such as an aortic aneurysm may impinge on the esophagus but will not usually appear as a fixed mass on fluoroscopy. Strictures caused by inflammation often involve more esophagus and present as a much longer segment of narrowing than carcinoma (Fig. 13-15). Varices may mimic carcinoma, but the linear defects are not fixed. They move as the patient swallows the barium (Fig. 16). Finally, moniliasis may mimic the mucosal appearance of carcinoma (Fig. 17), but is usually more diffuse in the esophagus. Wiot and Nelson make the key point that cineradiography of the barium swallow may be necessary to make the diagnosis because the barium may move down the esophagus so fast that more subtle lesions are missed. Repetitive viewing with slow motion and stop framing increase the accuracy of these more subtle studies. Finally, the impression of the radiologist should be taken into consideration, and if the diagnosis of carcinoma appears to be likely radiographically and biopsy is negative, repeat biopsy should be undertaken until the diagnosis is confirmed.

ENDOSCOPY AND BIOPSY

If the barium study confirms carcinoma the diagnosis must be proven by tissue diagnosis. More importantly, even if the clinical impression of carcinoma is not confirmed by the barium swallow, esophagoscopy and biopsy are mandatory. Tissue diagnosis is the crucial step in the diagnostic evaluation. In the past, the straight esophagoscope (Fig. 18) was utilized for endoscopy and biopsy, but because of its relatively short length, large size, and rigidity, the diagnostic accuracy was often only 50% at best (100). Also, the procedure involved general anesthesia and its attendant risks, the expense of an operating room, and carried a small but definite risk of esophageal perforation. Today the fiberoptic esophagogastroscope (Fig. 19) has improved the diagnostic accuracy to 95% (98). This flexible endoscope is able to evaluate the distal side of the lesion, especially the cardia of the stomach, with much better accuracy, and the scope is long enough to visualize the distal stomach as well. Finally, the procedure can be done in almost any location and under local anesthesia with an intravenous sedative as supplement. It is important to take multiple biopsies (a minimum of six to eight) including specimens from all four quadrants of the wall of the esophageal lesion. Biopsies should be taken beyond the proximal edge, since the tissue at the proximal edge is often bunched up normal mucosa caused by the growth of the tumor upward. It is particularly important to take multiple biopsies with the flexible scope because the biopsy forceps is much smaller than the biopsy forceps that can be used with the straight scope. Along with generous biopsy material, endoscopic brush cytologic specimens should be taken, especially if the lumen of the lesion is too small to pass the endoscope through to evaluate the distal edge of the lesion. According to Winawer et al. (101), the diagnostic accuracy of the brush cytology technique approaches 97%. In only one patient out of a series of 30 patients was the correct diagnosis not made by cytologic specimen. More importantly, in Winawer's series, the accuracy of diagnosis combining biopsy and brush cytology was 100%.

If biopsy and brush cytology are negative and the clinical suspicion of carcinoma is still present, repeat endoscopy with repeat biopsy and brush cytology is mandatory. If this still does not reveal carcinoma, exploratory laparotomy and/or thoracotomy may be necessary to confirm a highly suspicious diagnosis. Again, the most important determinant in eventual diagnosis of carcinoma of the gastroesophageal junction is a high index of suspicion and perseverance with diagnostic procedures until the tissue diagnosis is finally confirmed.

OTHER STUDIES

Bone scans and liver scans are not cost efficient in terms of routine preoperative tests. If the patient is symptomatic with bone pain, films of the area in question followed by a bone scan should be used to evaluate the possibility of metastatic disease. It may even be necessary to biopsy the bone lesion to document the existence of tumor, since bone scans may be positive on the basis of diseases other than metastases. If no symptoms are present a bone scan is not indicated. Liver scans are not done routinely because the accuracy of diagnosis is generally quite poor. Direct observation of the liver during abdominal exploration at the time of surgery is the best method for determining the presence and extent of liver metastases. It is important to understand that the presence of liver or bone metastases alone does not necessarily place a patient in the inoperable category, for resection is often the best palliation even if cure cannot be achieved.

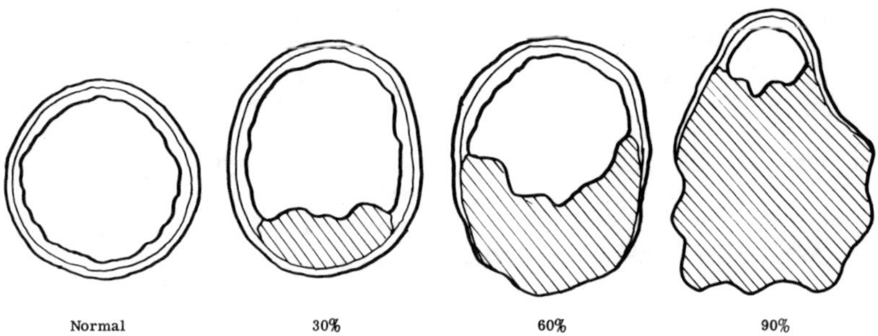

Figure 1: Because of the distensibility of the nonserosal covered esophageal wall, carcinoma must involve 75 to 90% of the circumference of the esophagus before obstruction occurs.

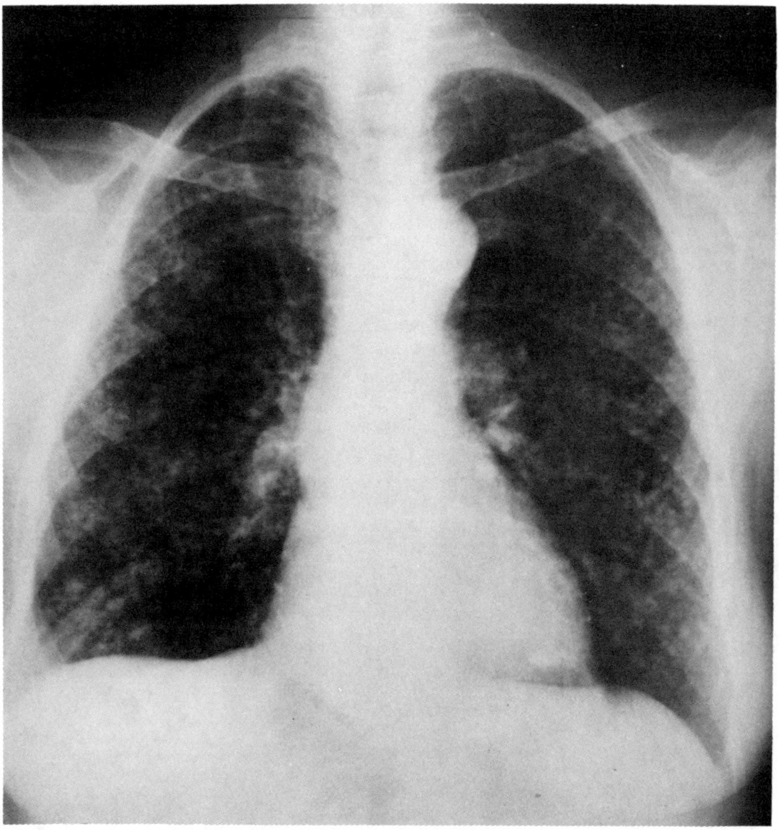

Figure 2: Carcinoma of the esophagus presenting with metastases to the lung.

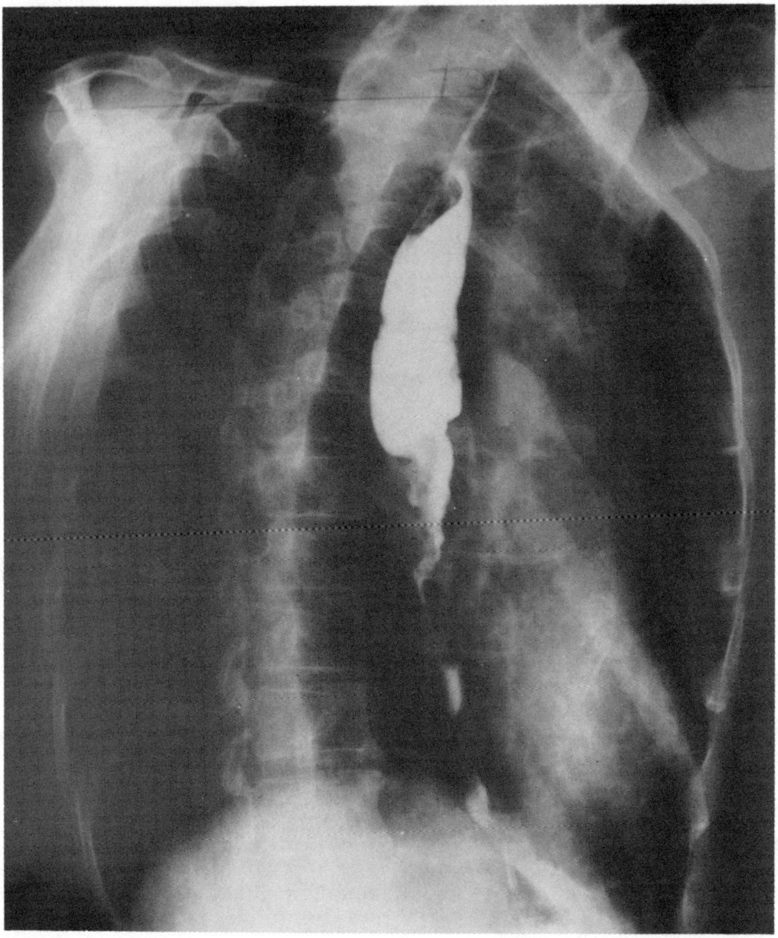

Figure 3: Squamous cell carcinoma of the esophagus, infiltrative type. Note the concentric narrowing of the lumen.

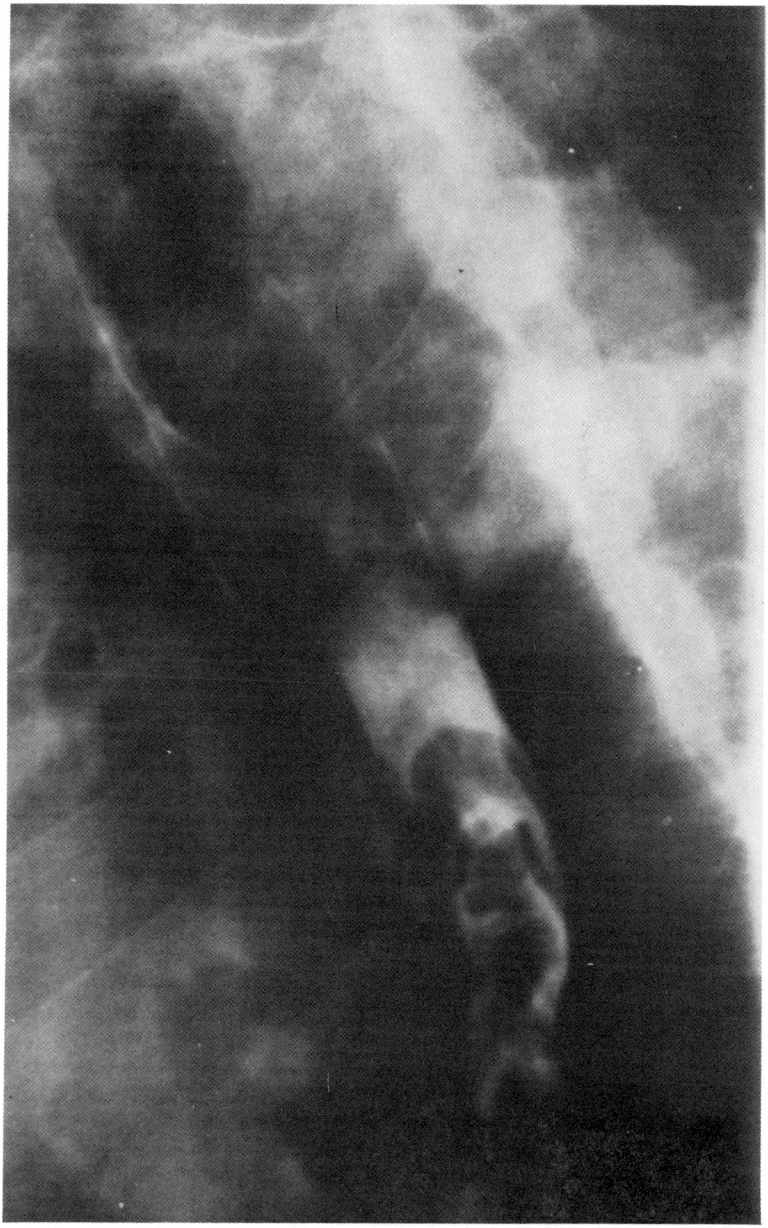

Figure 4: Carcinoma of the esophagus, polypoid form.

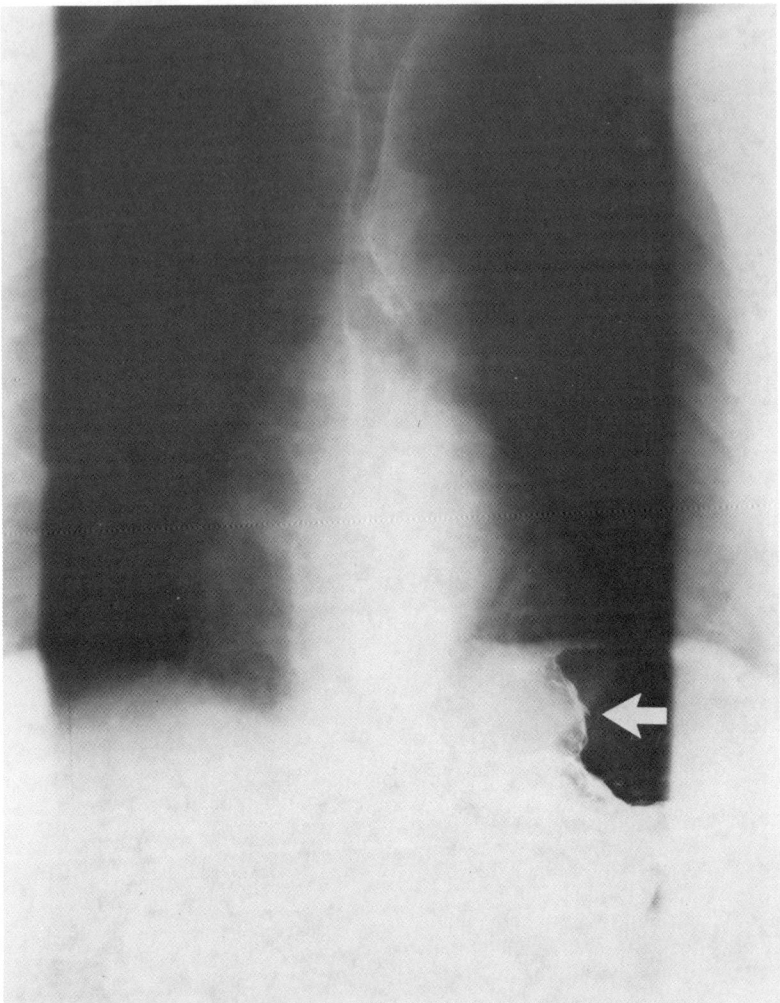

Figure 5: Squamous cell carcinoma of the gastroesophageal junction. Note the presence of the mass in the cardia (↑).

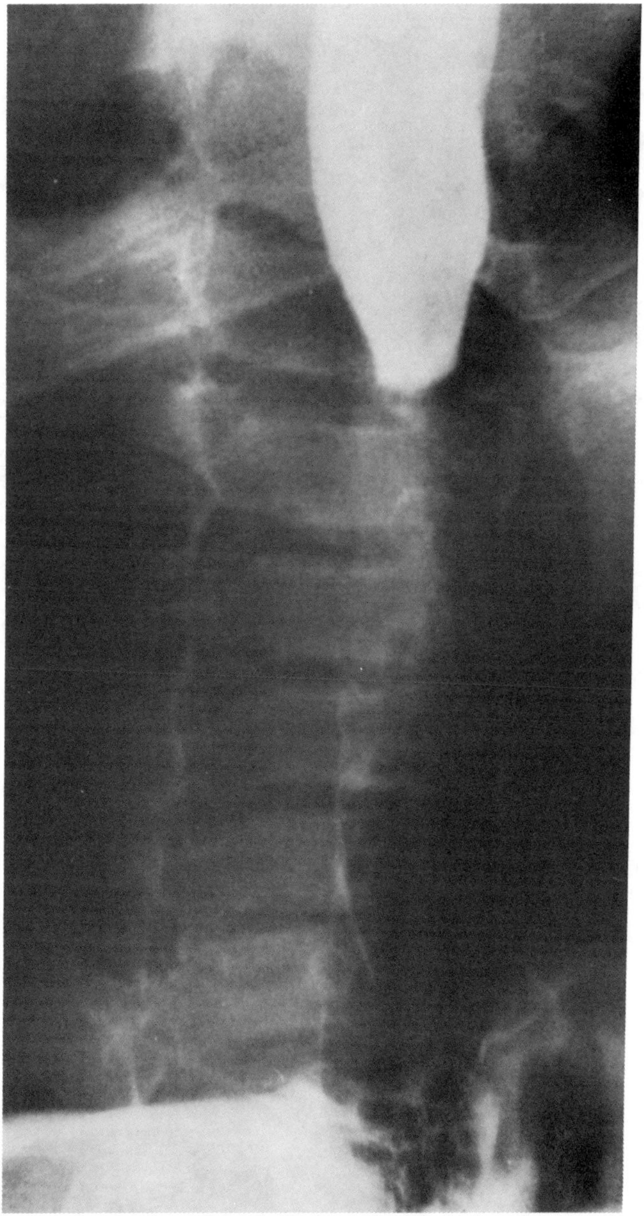

Figure 6: Complete occlusion of the esophagus secondary to carcinoma. The corner sign is present.

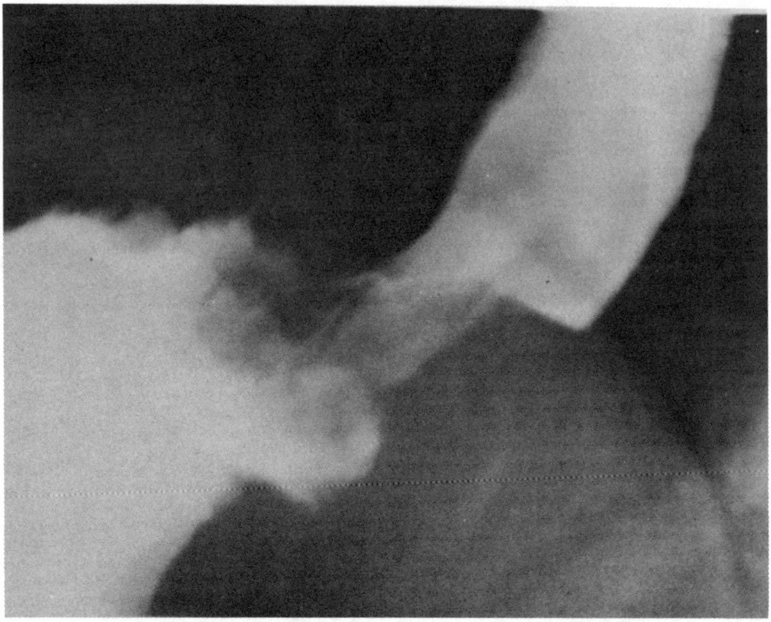

Figure 7: Carcinoma of the gastric cardia with classic step-off or corner sign.

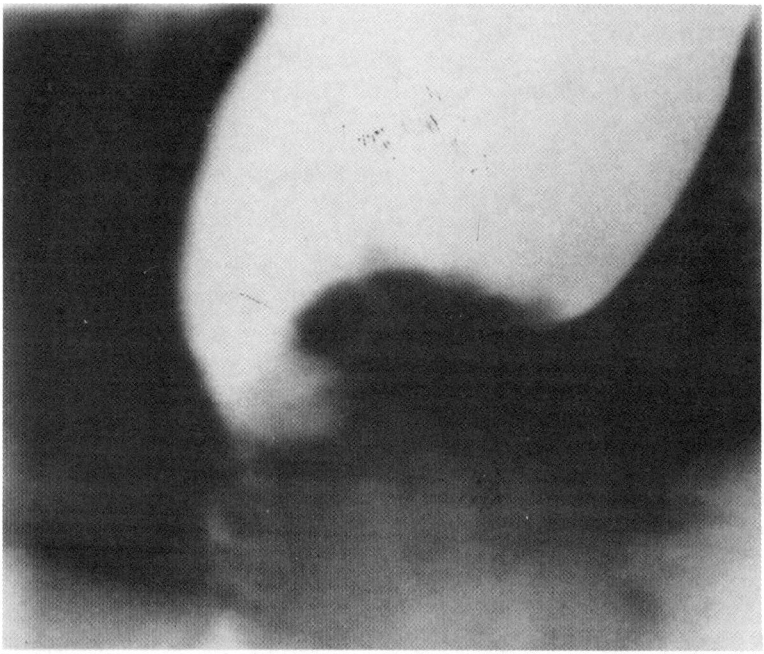

Figure 8: Carcinoma of the gastroesophageal junction with classic overhanging edge appearance of the proximal end of the tumor.

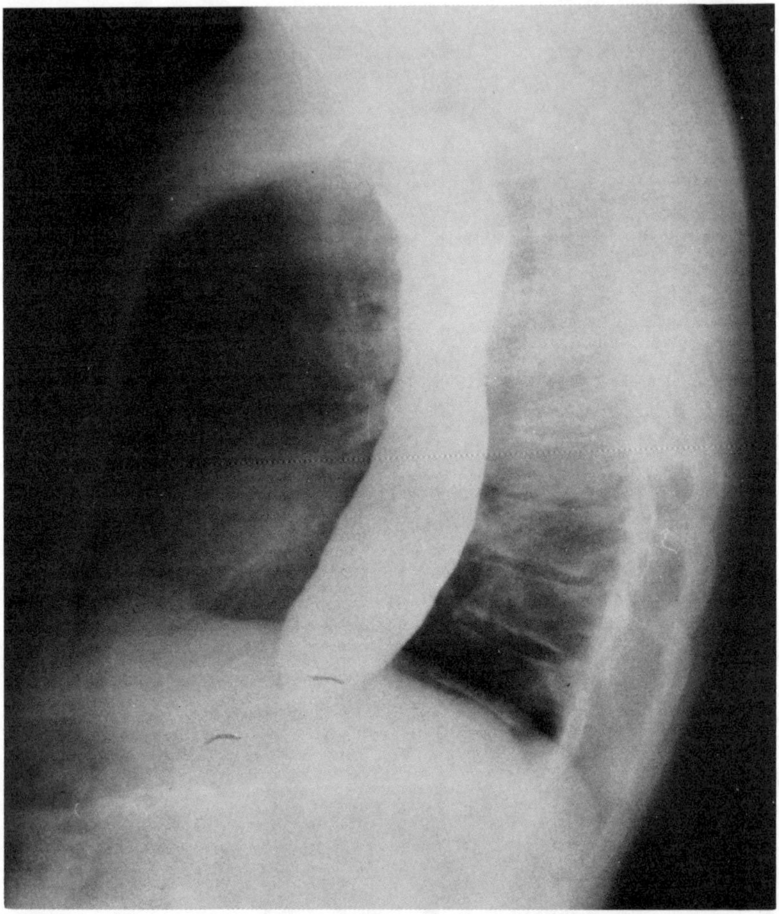

Figure 9: Achalasia: Note the dilated proximal esophagus which tapers smoothly to the narrowed distal esophagus. At fluoroscopy the area was nondistensible.

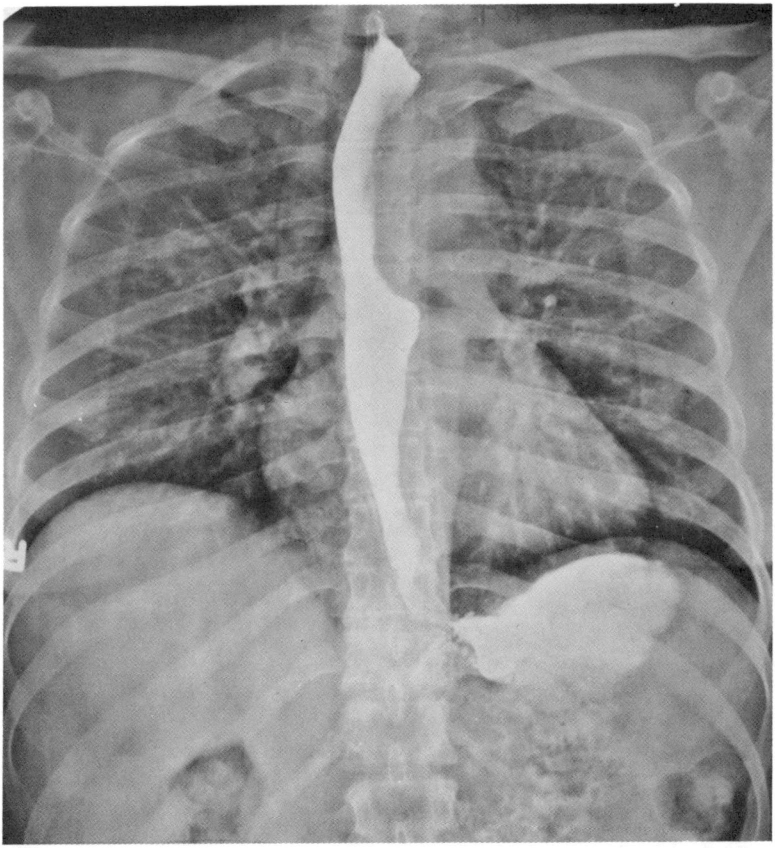

Figure 10: Intraluminal leiomyona. The barium swallow shows a filling defect of the upper esophagus with sharp borders suggesting an intraluminal lesion as opposed to either a mucosal or intrinsic mass.

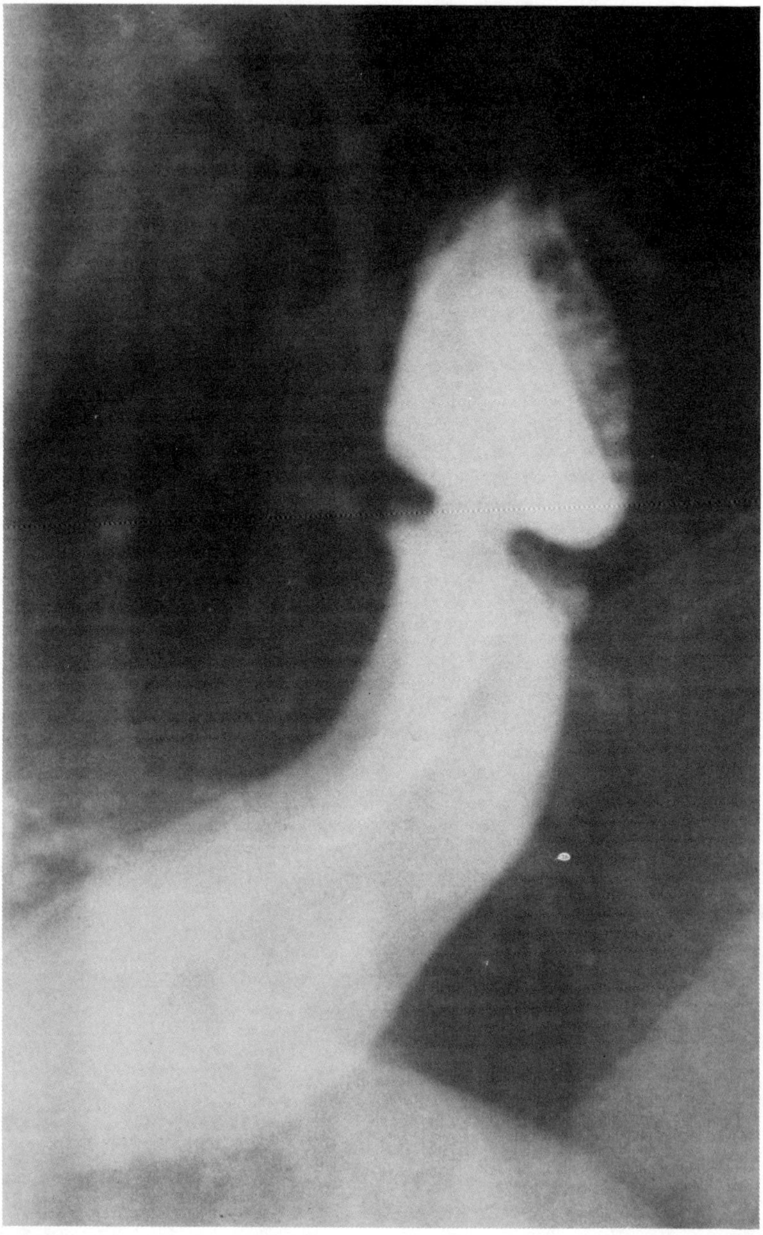

Figure 11: Schatzki's ring localized segment of distal esophagus with smooth edges indicating intact mucosa.

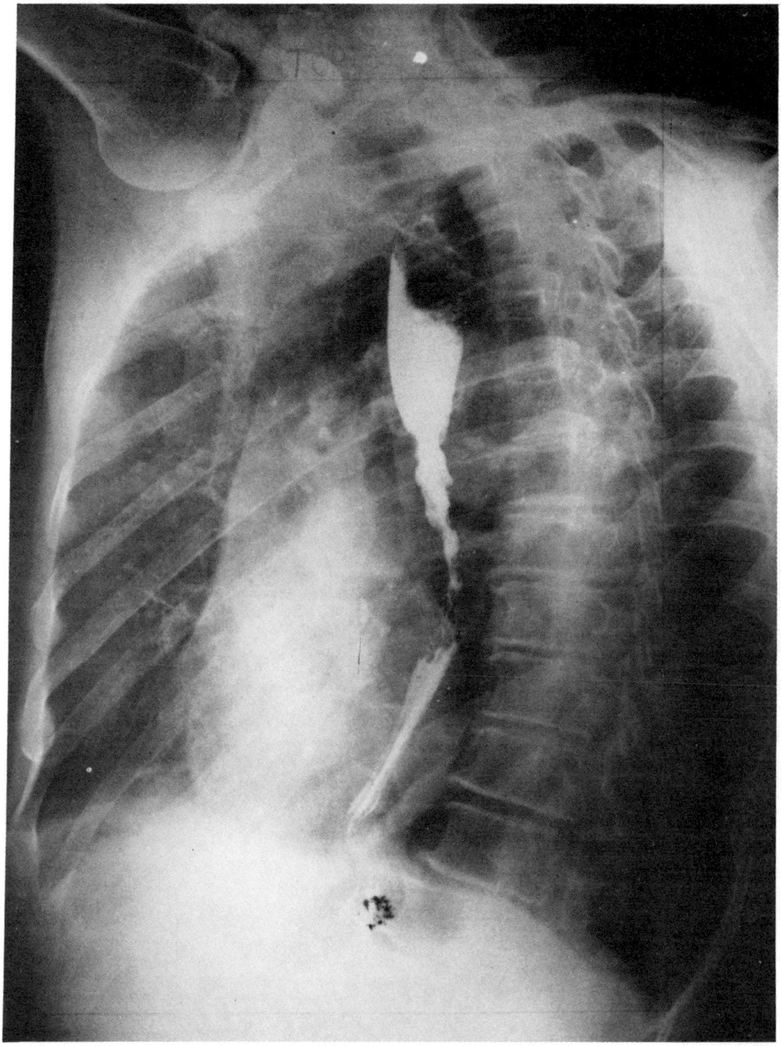

Figure 12: Infiltrating type carcinoma of the esophagus with shaggy mucosa indicating malignant disease.

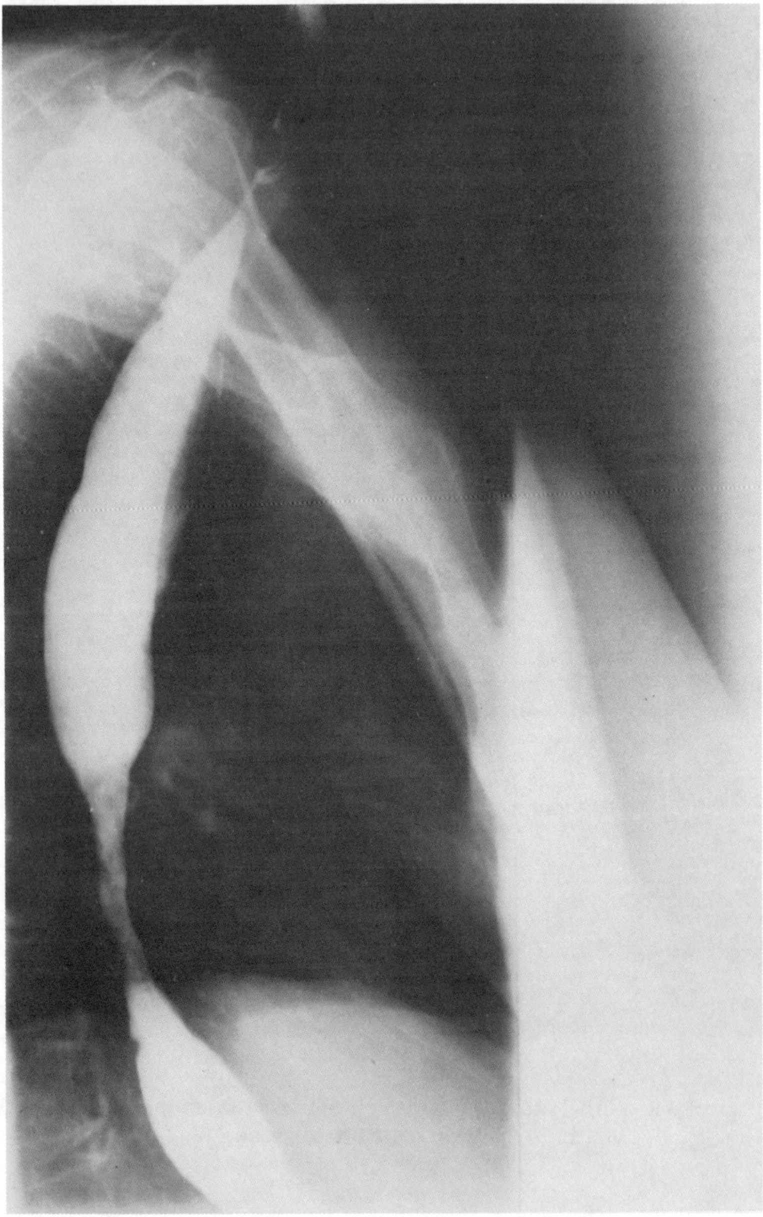

Figure 13: Scleroderma with distal esophageal stricture secondary to reflux. Note the proximal and distal tapering suggestive of benign disease.

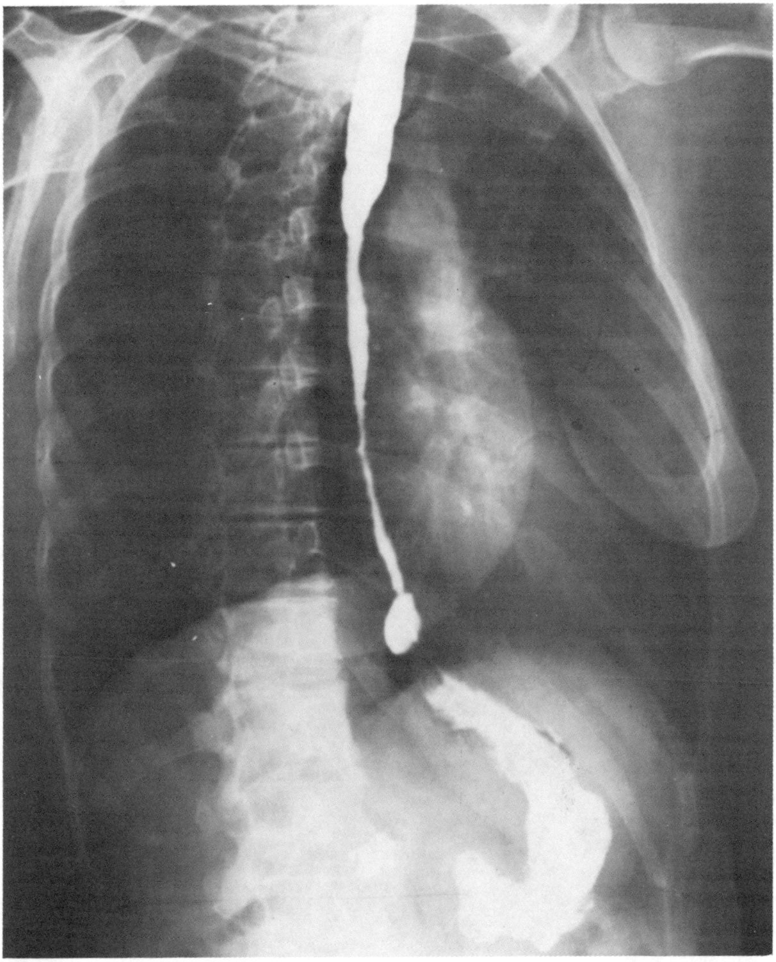

Figure 14: Dye ingestion with stricture. Note the length of the stricture. This is more suggestive of benign disease than carcinoma.

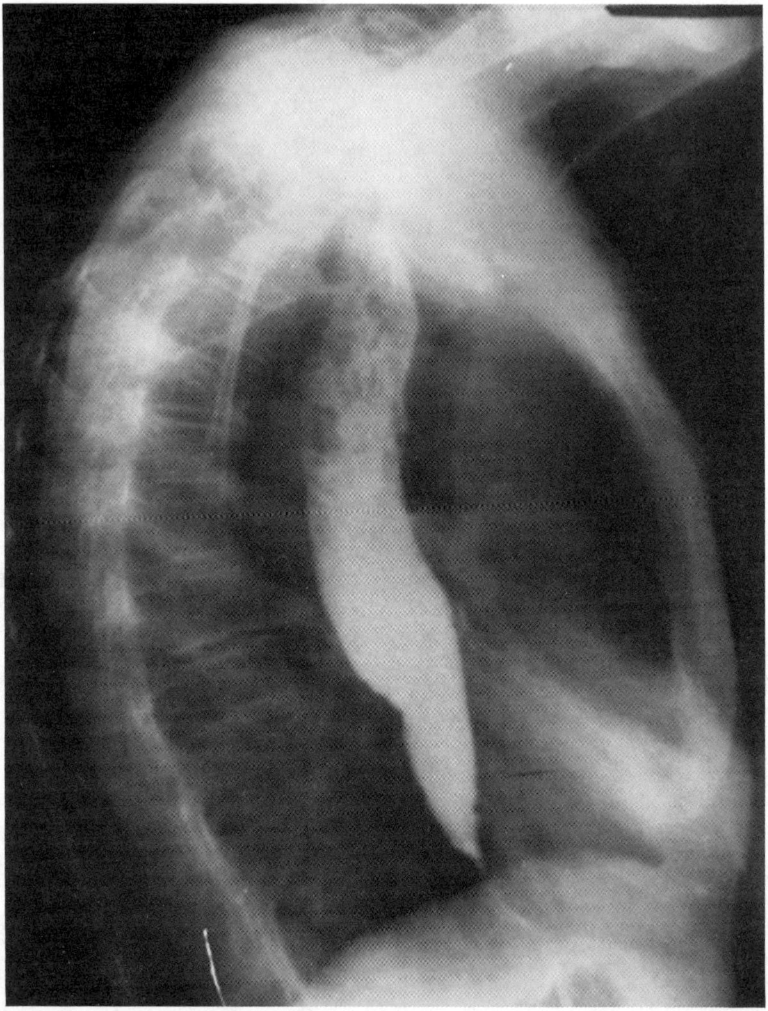

Figure 15: Tapering lesion of the distal esophagus initially felt to be benign stricture by the radiologist, but biopsy demonstrated carcinoma.

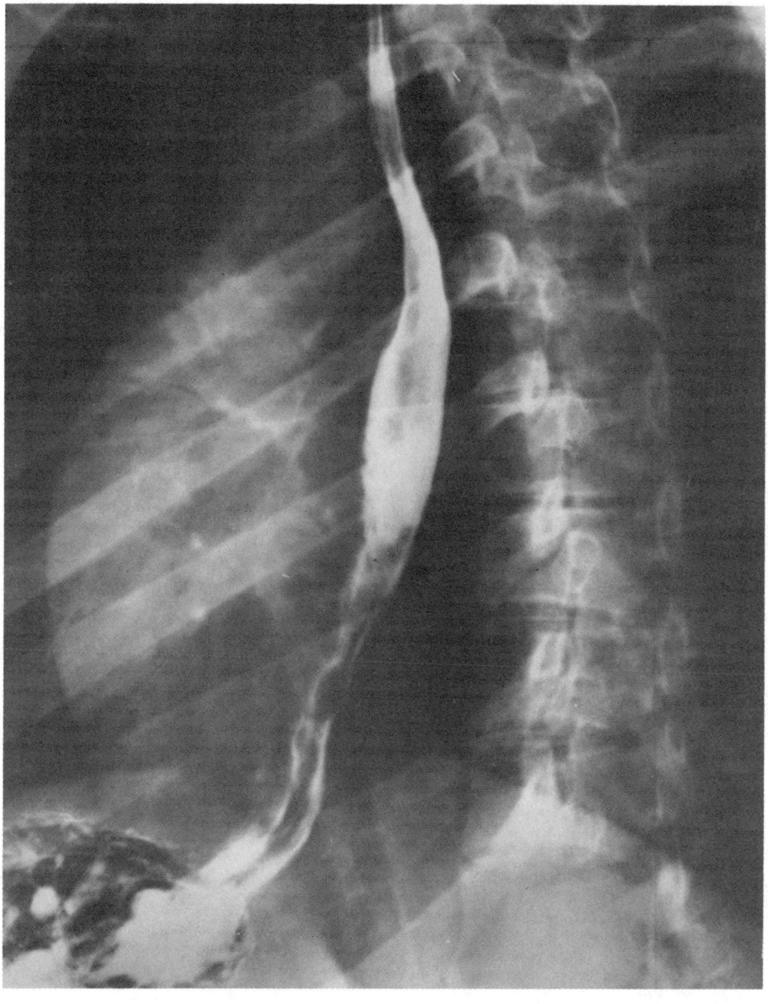

Figure 16A: Esophageal varice. This may be mistaken for carcinoma of the esophagus except that as the peristatic wave progresses, the varice will be obliterated.

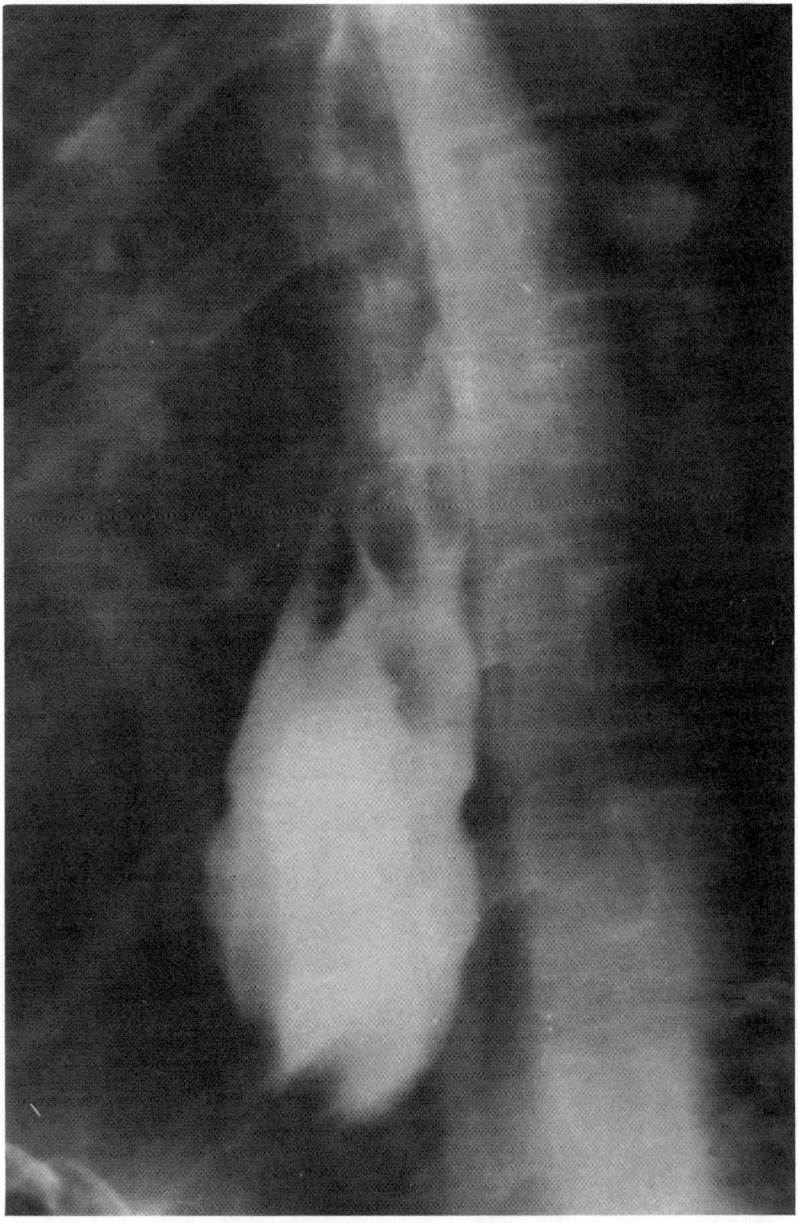

Figure 16B: Esophageal varice. This may be mistaken for carcinoma of the esophagus except that as the peristatic wave progresses, the varice will be obliterated.

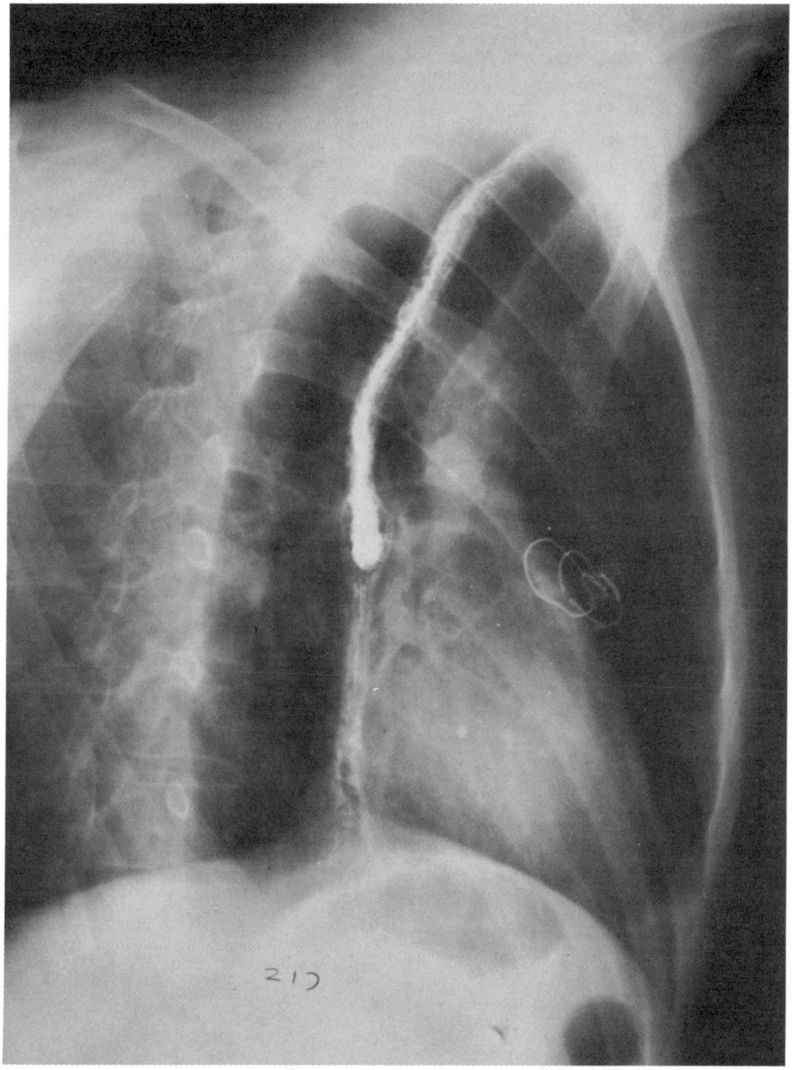

Figure 17: Moniliasis of the esophagus. Note the diffuse ragged pattern of the mucosa.

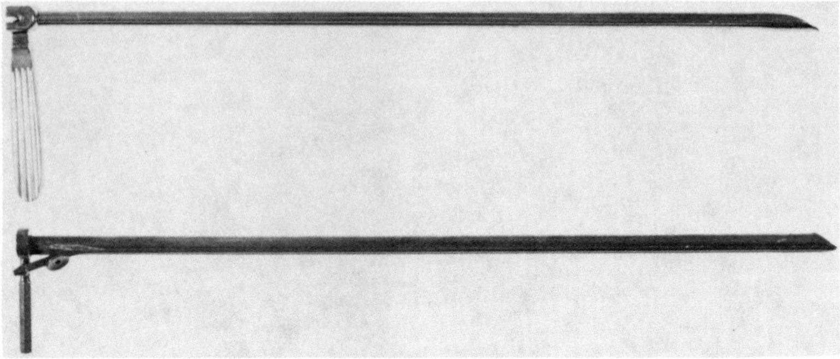

Figure 18: Jackson rigid esophagoscope below. Jesberg rigid esophagoscope above.

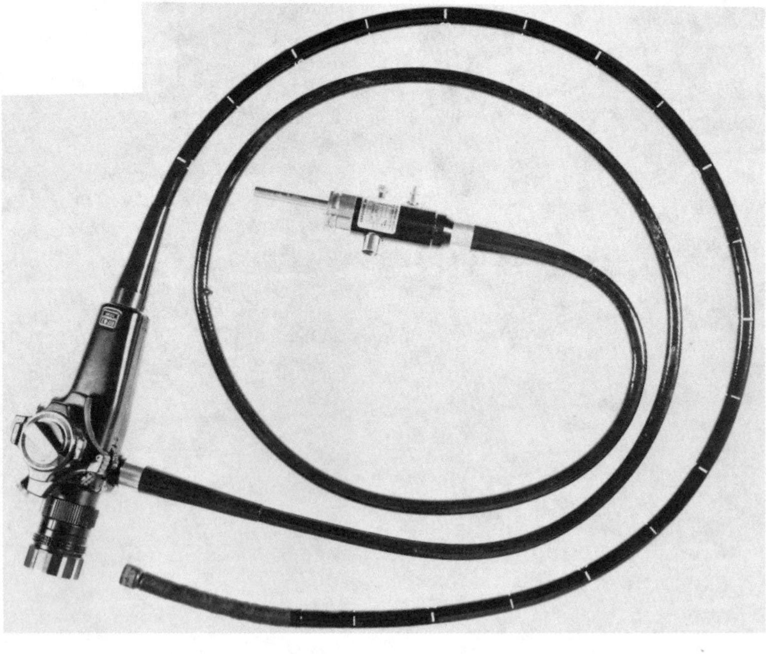

Figure 19: Olympus GIF-D_3 flexible fiberoptic esophagogastroscope.

Chapter 4

TREATMENT OF GASTROESOPHAGEAL CARCINOMA

GENERAL CONSIDERATIONS

In the earlier discussion of the pathophysiology of carcinoma of the gastroesophageal junction, the most striking feature about the course of this disease is that although the carcinoma probably remains localized for a significant period of time, the lesion is usually well advanced by the time clinical symptoms arise that alert the patient and his doctor of its presence. When the problem is finally appreciated and the patient has undergone the appropriate diagnostic studies, including a barium swallow and esophagoscopy to reveal a carcinoma of distal esophagus or gastroesophageal junction, the question of the appropriate therapy is dominated by three important factors: (1) the difficulty in clinically staging the extent of the disease prior to surgical intervention; (2) the need to palliate a very distressing symptom, e.g., the inability to swallow; and (3) the age of the patient, who is usually in the late 60s or early 70s when other disease processes and age often limit the scope of therapy.

Staging

As in all carcinomas, staging of esophageal carcinoma is best done according to the TNM system to assure uniformity. A close analysis of this system (Table 1 on page 12), however, reveals its limits when applied to the distal esophagus where examination of the regional lymph drainage, determination of the extent of the primary lesion, and the accurate examination of the most common sites of metastases require a significant surgical exploration.

Attempts at determining the invasiveness of the primary lesion by endoscopy are fraught with error. Although lesions which involve the full circumference and/or greater than 7 cm of length of the esophagus are more likely to be invasive into surrounding structures or metastatic to regional nodes, such lesions may also have remained relatively superficial in their invasion and localized in their spread. Immobility of the tumor (better assessed by rigid endoscopy as opposed to fiberoptic endoscopy) is an ominous sign of extraesophageal invasion of other structures best appreciated by an experienced esophagoscopist. Lesions that extend proximally to the level of the tracheal bifurcation should always undergo bronchoscopy, where the presence of visible tumor in the posterior wall of the trachea or main stem bronchi or fixation of the distal trachea (again better appreciated by rigid bronchoscopy) denotes invasion that is unresectable except in the most unusual circumstances. Lesions that on esophagoscopy show extensive involvement of the stomach tend to be further advanced, but again may only be superficially invasive. The extent of the lesion both proximally and distally as appreciated by endoscopy is crucial to planning any surgical resection.

A critical evaluation of the barium swallow is obviously valuable in determining the length of esophagus and stomach involved by the carcinoma. The esophageal involvement is usually fairly obvious, but special positioning and pressure manipulations of the abdomen may be necessary to fully evaluate the fundus and body of the stomach. The extent of invasion for staging purposes is not easily evaluated by barium swallow. Akiyama (102) has described a system of evaluating the esophageal axis on barium swallow which accurately predicts the extent of local invasion of the carcinoma (Fig. 20). In their retrospective analysis of 82 surgical cases of carcinoma of the esophagus, they found that none of 40 cases where a complete resection of the main lesion was possible had abnormalities of esophageal axis. In 12 patients where only a palliative resection was possible, 11/12 (91.7%) had abnormalities of esophageal axis. In 20 of the 30 patients who had exploration only because of unresectable disease there were abnormalities of esophageal axis. Overall in their experience, abnormalities of esophageal axis denoted invasiveness of the carcinoma beyond the limits of surgical resection. Most of their lesions were in the midesophagus, so there is concern that such definite statements about abnormalities of esophageal axis may be less accurate when applied to the esophagogastric junction where distortions of axis are more difficult to determine and if present may be less helpful in determining invasiveness.

Staging by mediastinoscopy may be helpful for squamous carcinoma of the cervical and upper thoracic esophagus but is not helpful in the evaluation of the distal esophagus or esophagogastric junction. Murray et al. (103) did routine mediastinoscopy in 30 patients with squamous cell carcinoma of the esophagus

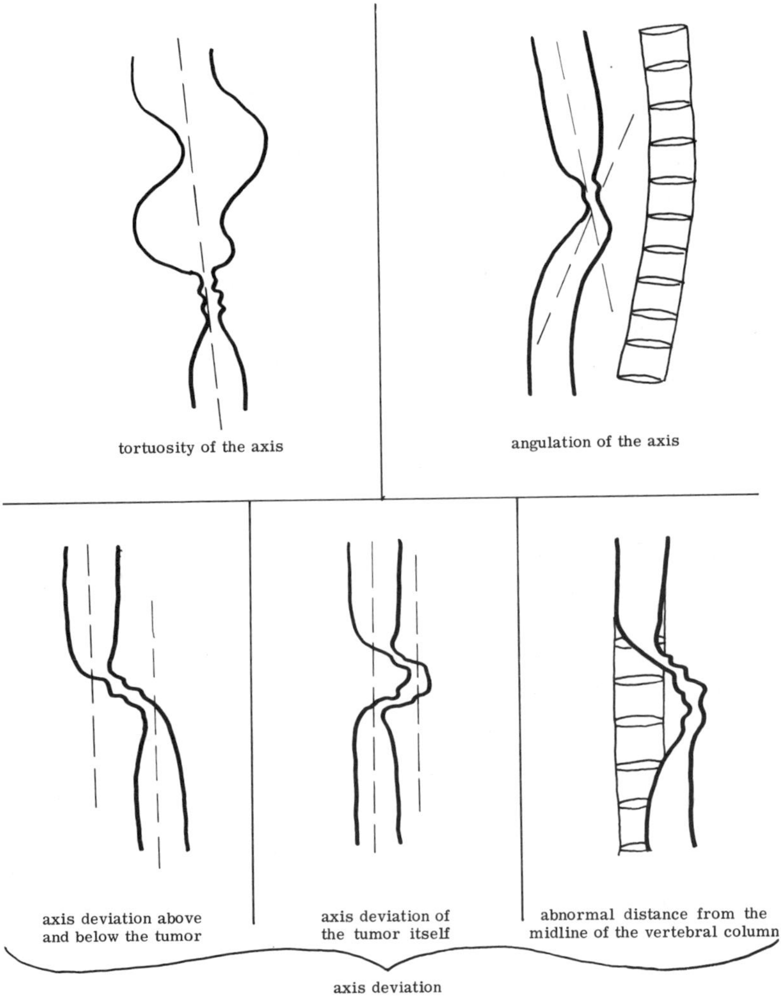

Figure 20: Abnormalities of esophageal axis denoting probable unresectability.

prior to surgical exploration. Ten of 18 patients with upper or midesophageal carcinoma had extraesophageal spread of cancer, and five of the ten (50%) were detected by mediastinoscopy. None of the 12 patients with lower esophageal carcinoma had positive mediastinoscopy; yet over one-half of the patients had extraesophageal spread of the cancer at the time of laparotomy or resection. Berglin et al. (104) also found mediastinoscopy inaccurate for staging squamous cell or adenocarcinoma of the distal esophagus and esophagogastric junction.

Liver scans are helpful only if grossly positive. Any positive or questionably positive liver scan must be confirmed by laparotomy since scan defects within the liver may be caused by other conditions, particularly cirrhosis of even mild to moderate degree, and apparent scan defects of edges of the liver may be due to anatomic variations alone. The liver scan can often be normal in the presence of multiple small metastases.

Liver function tests carry a similar significance to the liver scan. Elevations of serum bilirubin, SGOT, SGPT, and alkaline phosphatase may be present without liver metastases, or absent in the presence of liver metastases. As in metastases to the liver from any source, an elevation of alkaline phosphatase correlates better with metastases than any of the other liver function tests.

The new computerized axial tomography scan (CAT scan) of the mediastinum and abdomen is yet unproven in its value in staging carcinoma of the esophagus and stomach. Liver metastases are visualized well by this technique, possibly better than with the routine liver scan, but the presence of lymph node invasion can be misleading, as can the extent of local invasion by the primary tumor. Enlarged inflammatory nodes appear identical to enlarged metastatic nodes on CAT scan. A large primary carcinoma may appear to surround and invade the aorta on CAT scan, whereas at surgery there may be no invasion whatsoever. We have had more experience in the use of CAT scans to evaluate the mediastinum and local invasiveness of lung cancer where we have found it to be frequently misleading and inaccurate, usually by overestimating the extent of the disease.

Laparotomy has proven to be the most helpful procedure for staging carcinoma of the esophagus short of surgical resection. This is particularly true for carcinoma of distal esophagus and esophagogastric junction. Liver metastases, peritoneal seeding, the presence and extent of lymph node metastases, and in most instances of distal carcinomas, the extent of direct invasion of the primary carcinoma can all be evaluated by laparotomy. Squamous cell carcinoma of the distal esophagus and adenocarcinoma of the esophagogastric junction will usually first metastasize to nodes below the diaphragm, either the celiac nodes or the nodes along the short gastric vessels to the hilum of the spleen or tail of pancreas. The therapeutic alternatives based on the exploratory laparotomy will be discussed fully later.

In summary, because of the location of carcinoma of the distal esophagus and esophagogastric junction, the extent of local invasiveness, the presence or absence of regional lymph node invasion, and even the presence of more distant metastatic spread to liver and peritoneum can accurately be determined only by an exploratory laparotomy. Lesser procedures are inaccurate and misleading. Approximately 50 to 60% of these carcinomas, however, will reveal spread outside of the primary site making curative therapy an unlikely though possible goal. This high percentage of patients with advanced carcinoma should not dissuade us from seeking those patients with earlier lesions which are quite amenable to present therapy.

Palliation of Dysphagia

The dominant symptom in most patients with carcinoma of the esophagus is dysphagia, which if untreated usually leads to the total inability to swallow and to starvation months before death would otherwise occur from the metastatic spread of carcinoma. Only severe unrelenting pain, such as seen in invading carcinoma of the pancreas, progressive asphyxia as seen in end stage emphysemas or in obstructive tracheal tumors, are more distressing to the patient than the progressive inability to swallow. Any therapy of carcinoma of the esophagus and esophagogastric junction, regardless of the stage of the disease, which does not emphasize rapid and lasting palliation of dysphagia, is perceived by the patient as inadequate and by the doctor experienced in this disease as inappropriately meddlesome.

The ideal treatment regime, therefore, must be aimed at palliating the distressing dysphagia in all patients, yet providing an attempt at long-term control of the carcinoma in as many patients as possible within the realm of reasonable risk to the patient.

Advanced Age and Related Risk Factors

As mentioned in the section on the pathophysiology of carcinoma of the esophagogastric junction, the age of these patients is usually the late 60s and 70s. Advanced age, per se, does not contradict aggressive therapy of esophageal carcinoma. However, often coupled with the debility from their dysphagia, starvation, and often metastatic carcinoma, is further debility from chronic lung disease, coronary artery disease, peripheral vascular disease, cirrhosis, senility, previous surgery, and other problems of older age. All such problems must be evaluated closely to determine their influence in compounding the risk of each alternative form of therapy.

Chronic obstructive pulmonary disease (COPD) can be separated into three distinct parameters: (1) pure emphysema with overall loss of alveolar-capillary units; (2) chronic bronchitis with copious bronchial secretions and recurrent infection; and (3) asthma with episodic airway obstruction from hyperactive bronchial smooth muscle. In an individual patient with COPD one of these parameters may be dominant, but all are usually present in varying degrees.

Serious COPD can usually be suspected by the routine history and physical exam, but since lung function plays such an important role in the perioperative course in patients undergoing esophageal resection, we recommend routine measurement of the ventilatory functions of forced expiration volume (FEV) and the forced expiratory volume expired in the first second (FEV-1), and arterial blood gases (pH, pO_2, base excess), in addition to careful review of the chest X-ray and EKG to assess the degree of risk from chronic lung disease.

Chronic productive bronchitis should be treated with cessation of smoking, a ten-day course of appropriate antibiotics if the sputum cultures grow pathological organisms, and aggressive physical hygiene emphasizing postural drainage exercises, all over a two-week preoperative period. Asthmatic airway obstruction should be treated aggressively with bronchodilator medication. Aminophylline is particularly recommended because of the ability to give this drug either orally or parenterally during the perioperative period. When the patient's pulmonary function is maximized by these measures, repeat ventilatory functions and arterial blood gases should be obtained for truly accurate determination of the risk.

We generally estimate that an esophageal resection procedure will inflict an acute pulmonary compromise approximately equal to a pulmonary lobectomy with gradual recovery over two to three weeks. Radical esophageal radiation will inflict approxmately the same reduction of lung function gradually over several months due to the fibrosis of lung tissue in the ports of irradiation with the maximum deficit at about six months. With this expectation, analysis of pulmonary function tests are more accurate.

The most ominous signs of severe pulmonary compromise are retention of CO_2 and evidence of cor pulmonale on EKG and chest X-ray. Any rise in arterial pCO_2 above the normal of 40 mmHg denotes increased risk, and a rise to 50 or greater denotes prohibitive risk for either esophageal resection or radical irradiation. If significant cor pulmonale is suspected on EKG and chest X-ray a more accurate determination of the risk can be obtained by a right heart catheterization with measurement of pulmonary artery pressure and pulmonary vascular resistance at rest and with exercise (105). Elevations of pulmonary vascular resistance which remains elevated with exercise denotes prohibitive risk.

The ventilation function tests of FEV and FEV-1 are not as precisely indicative of risk, but if the patient clinically appears to have significant pulmonary compromise and the FEV and/or FEV-1 is less than 40% of predicted, esophageal resection is prohibited and radical radiation is risky.

Heart disease is common in these aged patients with esophageal carcinoma, particularly ischemic heart disease, congestive heart failure, and occasionally valvular heart disease.

Ischemic heart disease carries a very identifiable risk (106-109). The mere presence of angina or history of a previous myocardial infarction adds 5 to 15% mortality risk to a significant operative procedure. The interval over which a previous infarction occurred is very important, with 40% mortality risk within three months of infarction decreasing to 5 to 10% after six months. Our policy is not to operate within three months of an acute myocardial infarction except in unusual circumstances, and to aggressively treat angina preoperatively with propranolol and nitrates which are continued through the procedure and in the postoperative period, giving these medications intravenously as indicated by very careful monitoring of arterial blood pressure, pulmonary artery wedge pressure, and cardiac output.

The risk of congestive heart failure in noncardiac surgery has been well documented and correlated to the New York Heart Association functional classification as follows (109):

NYHA Class	Operative Mortality
I	4%
II	11%
III	25%
IV	67%

We do not recommend esophageal resection in NYHA class IV (congestive heart failure symptomatic at rest). In classes II and III, digoxin and diuretic therapy are maximized preoperatively and continued through the postoperative period.

A helpful multifactorial index of cardiac risk in noncardiac operations has been proposed by Goldman et al. (108) based on nine parameters and four classes:

1)	Age > 70	5 points
2)	Acute MI in previous six months	10 points
3)	Presence of S_3 gallop or jugular venous distension	11 points
4)	Significant valvular aortic stenosis	3 points
5)	Rhythm other than sinus	7 points
6)	Greater than five ventricular ectopic beats/minute	7 points
7)	Poor general medical condition	3 points
8)	Intraperitoneal, thoracic, or aortic procedure	3 points
9)	Emergency operation	4 points

Class	Points	Serious Cardiac Morbidity	Cardiac Mortality
I	0-5	0.7%	0.2%
II	6-12	5.0%	2.0%
III	13-25	11.0%	2.0%
IV	>25	22.0%	56.0%

Under this scheme, class IV patients should not undergo significant operative procedures.

With the exception of carotid artery disease, the presence of peripheral artery disease, unless very severe, does not seem to add appreciable risk to esophageal resection. The presence of a critical stenosis of a carotid artery does carry significant risk of stroke in the perioperative period, so our policy is to do angiography on all patients with symptomatic carotid artery disease and at least plethysmography on asymptomatic carotid bruits preoperatively. If a severely stenotic carotid artery is identified, carotid endarterectomy is done prior to esophageal surgery. Mild to moderate stenosis or ulcerated plaques are not considered indications for surgical treatment prior to esophageal resection. In the presence of other signs of peripheral vascular disease, consideration must be given to possible involvement of the intestinal blood supply which could affect the organ used for esophageal replacement. This problem will be considered later.

The presence of severe cirrhosis, especially with portal hypertension, is generally a contraindication to esophageal resection because of the prohibitive risk of liver failure and/or severe bleeding from the extensive dissection. Abnormalities of liver function, particularly depressed serum albumin and prothrombin time and the typical physical findings of ascites, spider angioma, and collateral venous channels, are helpful in identifying these patients.

Previous surgical procedures may influence the choice of surgical therapy. Previous gastric surgery generally does not preclude an esophagogastrectomy but may necessitate replacement by jejunum or colon. Previous abdominal aortic surgery, pancreatitis, or colectomy may have left enough adhesions to interfere with esophagogastrectomy. Previous pulmonary surgery may make the thoracic exposure difficult. All must be considered before the decision for esophagogastrectomy.

Neither diabetes nor hypertension seem to carry an appreciable risk to major surgery if their presence is recognized preoperatively and appropriate monitoring and therapy are exercised.

SELECTION OF THERAPY FOR CARCINOMA OF THE LOWER ESOPHAGUS AND ESOPHAGOGASTRIC JUNCTION

Several modes of therapy have been advocated for carcinoma of the lower esophagus and cardia with varying degrees of success in terms of cure rates and palliation.

Radiation Therapy

As a primary form of therapy, radiation for carcinoma of the esophagus and particularly the lower esophagus and cardia has generally had only limited success. Most authors report few long-term survivors after radiation therapy for carcinoma of the esophagus. Watson (110) reviewed 672 patients treated with various techniques of radiation therapy and found only seven long-term survivors (1% five-year survival).

Wilson (111) compared radiation (5800 r over six to eight weeks) to surgical resection in 20 comparable patients of each group with carcinoma of the midesophagus and found no long-term survivors in the radiation group versus 15% long-term survival in the surgical group. Moreover, only 20% of the radiation group was able to swallow a normal diet versus 90% of the surgical group. The common mode of death in the radiation group was aspiration pneumonitis, whereas most of the surgical patients died of generalized metastases. Friedman (112) also noted only rare survival after radical radiation for carcinoma of the esophagus. Pearson (113-116) remains the chief advocate for radiation as the primary choice of therapy for carcinoma of the esophagus. In his series of 720 patients treated in Edinburgh for squamous carcinoma of the esophagus between 1949 and 1967, he noted an increase in survival in the patients treated with radical radiation versus the patients treated with surgical resection. The overall five-year survival in the radiated group was 48/288 (17%) versus 48/432 (11%) for the surgical group. Radiation consisted of 5000 r of orthovoltage X-rays using two opposed fields over a five-week period. His results with squamous carcinoma of the lower esophagus showed equal five-year survivals in radiated and resected patients (12/103 or 12% for radiated patients versus 32/281 or 11% for surgical patients). There are two criticisms of Pearson's study. A number of patients were included in the study without histological proof of carcinoma (113). Since all surgical patients would have eventual histological verification of carcinoma, these patients with an uncertain diagnosis would primarily bias the radiation group. Many patients receiving palliative radiation (113) were not included in the analysis without clearly demonstrating that the initial intent of the radiation in each of these patients was indeed palliative and not curative. Both of these factors would tend to favor the results in the radiation treated group. Interestingly, surgery is presently favored over radiation for carcinoma of the esophagus in Edinburgh (117). Rider (118) has shown that the technique and dose of radiation therapy is crucial to satisfactory results. He had no long-term survivals if the dose was less than 4000 r in four weeks or greater than 6000 r in six weeks; whereas, doses of 4500 r in four weeks and 6000 r in six weeks gave a five-year survival of 10 to 20%.

Although radiation is favored over surgical resection in carcinoma of the upper and midesophagus by many authors (114, 116, 119, 120), only Pearson (116) favors radiation for treatment for squamous carcinoma of the distal esophagus, and radiation is generally not advocated for adenocarcinoma of the esophagogastric junction. Surgical resection of distal one-third squamous carcinoma gives five-year survival of 20 to 30% (2, 75, 203); whereas, in the most favorable study, Pearson (116) reports only 12% survival at five years for radiation therapy. Decreased response to radiation in the lower esophagus and cardia with both squamous and adenocarcinoma has generally been attributed to the larger volumes of tissue that must be treated in order to include these tumors and their regional lymph drainage. Adenocarcinoma at the esophagogastric junction has generally been considered poorly responsive to radiation therapy; however, Humphrey (121), in reporting the results of therapy in 592 patients with carcinoma of the distal esophagus and cardia, noted superior long-term survival with surgical resection in patients with both squamous and adenocarcinoma as opposed to radiation therapy, but equal palliation of adenocarcinoma versus squamous carcinoma when treated with radiation therapy.

Nonresolution or return of dysphagia after radiation for carcinoma of the esophagus and cardia is relatively common and is most often due to either recurrent carcinoma or fibrous stricture. In Pearson's study (113) only 59/144 (41%) patients returned to a normal diet and 39/144 (27%) required bougienage. Relief of dysphagia after radiation is usually delayed for several weeks after therapy. Some degree of pulmonary fibrosis in the radiated field invariably occurs after radical radiation therapy, which in our experiences generally corresponds functionally to the loss of approximately 20 to 25% of functional lung gradually over a six-month period. Rarely osteitis of the vertebral bodies (113) or constrictive pericarditis (122) have developed after radiation for carcinoma of the esophagus.

Radiation Combined with Surgical Resection

The use of preoperative radiation as an adjuvant of surgical resection for carcinoma of the esophagus has been advocated by Nakayama and Akakura in Japan, and Parker in the United States.

Nakayama's reports (123, 124) cover patients who were treated with a three-stage operative procedure for resection of carcinoma of the esophagus in conjunction with preoperative radiation. The first stage was an exploratory celiotomy with biopsy of celiac nodes and gastrostomy. Patients without significant metastases were given 2000 to 2500 r of radiation over four to five days. The second stage was total thoracic esophagectomy through the right chest 10 to 14 days after radiation. The third stage was completed after the patient had gained nutrition by connecting the cervical esophagostomy to the gastrostomy by a rubber tube and consisted of a subcutaneous stomach tube anastamosed to the cervical esophagus. Of 200 patients who completed this entire treatment regime, there was a 2.5% operative mortality. Of those with upper and midesophageal lesions there was a four-year survival of 31.8% and five-year survival of 37.5%,* compared to previous series which had shown four-year and five-year survivals of 15.4% and 19.1% respectively for patients treated by resection alone, and 6.3% and 7.7% respectively for patients undergoing only radiation. No mention is made in these reports of the long-term results with carcinoma of the distal esophagus and cardia, and severe criticism of the reports is centered on the lack of information about the number of patients who were begun on this treatment regime but deleted from the final statistics because of failure to complete the entire course of therapy.

---

* Some patients followed for four years had not yet been followed for five years so that the calculated five-year survival data exceeded the four-year survival, a statistical anomaly that can occur if all patients have not been followed for the five-year period.

Akakura (125) compared surgical resection alone in 229 patients to preoperative radiation combined with surgical resection in 117 patients. Radiation consisted of 5000 to 6000 r over 30 to 40 days and was followed in two to four weeks by one stage esophagogastrectomy. Operative mortality in the preoperative radiation group was 20.8% compared to 13.2% in the group with surgical resection only. The five-year survival was 25% in the preoperative radiation group and 13.6% in the surgical group. All of these carcinomas were squamous cell in histological type and no separation in results is discussed regarding lower esophageal carcinomas.

Parker (126-128), noting very poor results from surgery (0.6% two-year survival) before 1951 and radiation alone (5% two-year survival) from 1951 to 1957, began a treatment regime of preoperative radiation with 4500 r over four weeks followed by surgical excision in all squamous carcinomas of the esophagus treated between 1957 and 1967. If surgical excision was not possible for any reason, the radiation was carried to 6000 r. Ninety-one out of 138 patients were deemed inoperable with six two-year and three five-year survivals. Forty-seven out of 138 patients underwent resection after radiation with 11 two-year and nine five-year survivals. Overall two-year survival was 12% and five-year survival was 8.7%. On the basis of these results compared to their previous experience, Parker advocates preoperative radiation therapy. Again, adenocarcinomas are not included and results with distal esophageal carcinomas are not reported separately.

In each of these reports a high incidence of residual carcinoma has been noted in the operative specimens after the preoperative radiation (87.5% in Parker's series) (128).

Groves (129) reports a series of 70 patients with carcinoma of the esophagus and cardia with approximately one-half of the patients having adenocarcinoma. Preoperative radiation consisted of 2400 r in three days followed in 10 to 14 days by esophagogastrectomy. All five long-term survivors were patients without positive nodes. Groves' conclusion was that there was no benefit to preoperative radiation and he no longer uses this approach.

Although there is some suggestion that preoperative radiation is effective, all of these reports use historical controls for comparison, and only Groves addresses both squamous and adenocarcinoma of the distal esophagus and cardia. Our own small experience with preoperative radiation has led us to abandon this combination of therapy because of a high incidence of pulmonary complications, which we believe is attributable to the surgical stress of thoracotomy and lung retraction on the preexisting radiation lung injury. We have rarely seen this major pulmonary failure after resection alone.

Several authors favor prophylactic postoperative radiation after resection of esophageal carcinoma. Fraser (130) studied the results of immediate sequential radiation therapy (either pre- or postoperative) combined with surgical resection. Of eight patients who received radiation postoperatively, two patients had radiation immediately postoperatively for microscopic tumor in the resection margin and both lived ten years. Five of eight patients had delayed radiation after tumor recurrence with no long-term survivors. Kasai (131) reported an overall five-year survival rate of 16.5% after resection of carcinoma of the esophagus, but a 34.6% five-year survival in patients who received prophylactic postoperative radiation and 87.5% five-year survival in prophylactic postoperative radiation in patients who did not have lymph node metastases.

Surgical Resection

The published results of several major series of patients undergoing surgical resection for carcinoma of the distal esophagus and cardia are discussed in a later section and are summarized in Table 6.

In large series, five-year survival rates are 20 to 30%. Palliation of dysphagia is generally excellent with less than 20% of the operative survivors having return of dysphagia. The main deterrent to surgical resection remains the immediate high operative mortality which has previously been reported to be 15 to 30%. With more careful attention to operative detail and perioperative care this mortality is falling progressively and now is generally accepted at 5 to 10% for resection of distal esophagus and cardia. Dysphagia is relieved rapidly and hospitalization is generally limited.

Because the results have been good in comparison to radiation alone or preoperative radiation plus resection, our practice has been to plan a radical surgical resection on all appropriate patients as outlined in the Selective Therapy Scheme (Table 2). Only rarely do we employ radiation therapy for curative treatment, reserving its use to situations when there are overwhelming medical contraindications to operation in patients with seemingly localized disease. Our indications for postoperative radiation therapy are limited to the presence of microscopically positive nodes or malignant tissue at or near the resection margins when all other evidence of carcinoma has been removed. In those circumstances 5000 r are focused on the worrisome areas in a five-week course.

Table 2 Selective Therapy Scheme

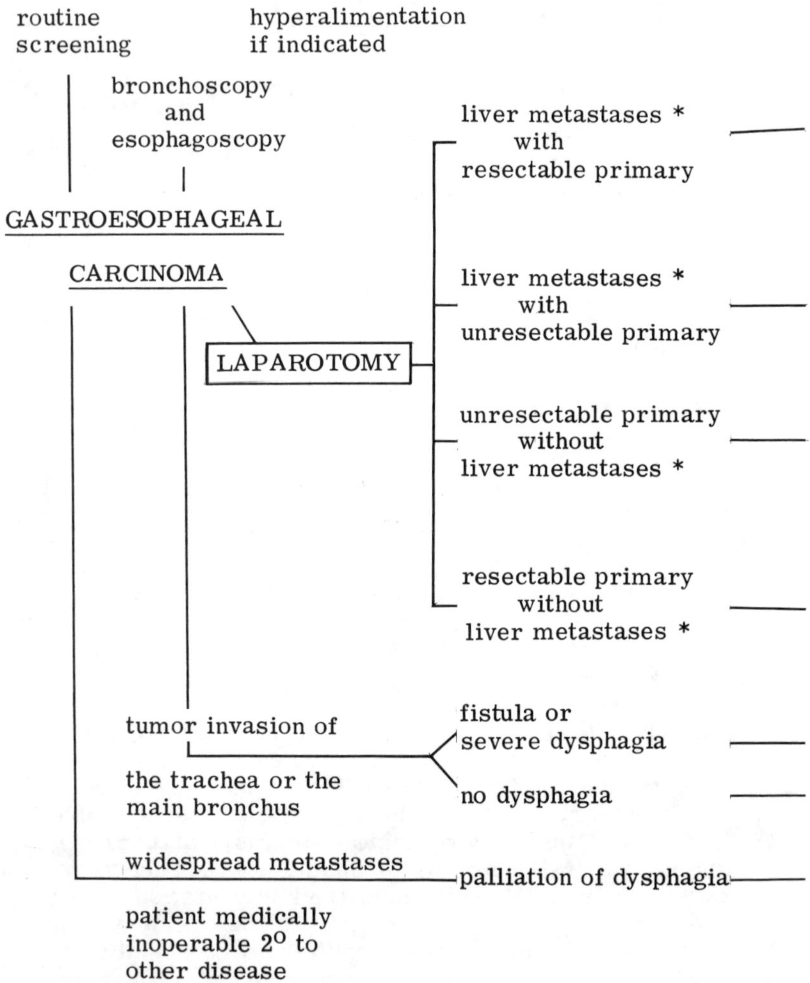

* or peritoneal seeding of tumor

- dysphagia significant
  1. limited resection
  2. Celestin tube intubation
- dysphagia not significant
  1. no resection
  2. later palliation as needed with pulsion tube or radiation

1. Celestin tube intubation
2. limited bypass
3. radiation to the primary

1. colon bypass followed by radical radiation if no metastases or only local node metastases
2. colon bypass alone
3. Celestin tube intubation

- (+) nodes outside resection margin — limited resection
- (+) nodes within resection margin / (-) nodes — radical esophago-gastrectomy
- extensive stomach involvement — radical esophago-gastrectomy with total gastrectomy

— pulsion tube intubation

— no therapy (especially no radiation)

- pulsion tube intubation
  or
  radiation of the primary

Palliation as the Only Therapy

In many circumstances where curative therapy is inappropriate, palliation of the severe dysphagia is the only desired treatment. Several modes of palliation are available.

Feeding Gastrostomy

Feeding gastrostomy is mentioned only to condemn its use except in circumstances where the physician may wish to provide temporary nutrition as a step in a more elaborate treatment regime. As a simple palliative procedure, a feeding gastrostomy does not provide for the patient the ability to chew and swallow his meals and eventually does not even allow the patient to swallow his own saliva. The great tendency toward aspiration and pneumonitis are not relieved. The only palliation is some increased nutrition. Dickison (132) observed the fates of 55 patients with inoperable carcinoma who had palliative gastrostomy as opposed to 23 similar patients who had palliative radiation or no therapy. In the patients with gastrostomy, 42% died in the hospital without discharge, and the average survival was 120 days. The patients without gastrostomy had an average survival of 111 days. He concluded that gastrostomy did not prolong life and did not actually palliate but only added misery to the majority. King (133) analyzed 29 gastrostomies for incurable cancer and found only six of 29 who were considered to have had an acceptable response (not measurably harmed by the procedure). In these six good responders the average survival was only four and one-half months. Eight of 29 patients died in the hospital within 30 days, and five of 29 additional patients were clearly harmed by the procedure. The gastrostomy wounds healed poorly and often opened a route for serious infection. Our own experience has been very similar. The death and complication rate is extremely high and adequate oral alimentation which the patient perceives as good palliation is not achieved.

Simple Dilatation

Simple dilatation of inoperable carcinoma of the esophagus using Maloney, Eder-Puestow, or Hurst dilators has been advocated by Heit (134), for palliation of dysphagia. Six hundred and sixteen dilatations were done on 26 patients. Twenty-three of 26 patients were also receiving radiation therapy to the primary lesion during the period of dilatations and four of 26 patients had dilatation prior to prosthetic intubation of the esophagus, so there is considerable question as to the relative role of the dilatations in relief of dysphagia. Twenty-four of 26 patients were able to resume a soft or regular diet and there was only one serious complication, a closed perforation which did not require operation. Dilatation alone is not recommended, since the carcinoma invariably grows back to cause recurrent dysphagia, but is often useful as an adjuvant to radiation or palliative intubation.

Prosthetic Intubation

Prosthetic intubation of the esophagus has a long history of use in the palliation of advanced carcinoma of the esophagus. Numerous types of tubes have been used over the years with favor swinging from a pulsion type tube (such as the original Souttar tube where the tube is pushed through the malignant obstruction in the esophagus) to a traction type tube (such as the Mousseau-Barbin tube which was later refined to the Celestin tube where the tube is pulled to a position bridging the malignant obstruction by first introducing a thin tube or rod through the tumor from above and out a gastrotomy incision). These traction type tubes offered a much larger lumen which allowed better palliation of swallowing. They suffered from the disadvantages of requiring laparotomy for the gastrotomy and anchoring of the tube within the stomach and of bridging the esophagogastric junction, leading to frequent reflux back into the esophagus. More recently there has been a resurgence of interest in larger pulsion type tubes such as the Palmer tube and the Proctor-Livingstone tube which require dilatation of the tumor before insertion, but which avoid a laparotomy. Because of the limited palliation of swallowing provided by the rigid tubes, the occasional migration of the tube above or below the tumor, and the frequent complications associated with their insertion, prosthetic tubes for palliation have generally been limited to use in unresectable carcinomas of the esophagus and cardia where the life expectancy is very limited and to palliative bridging of malignant tracheoesophageal fistulas.

The Celestin* tube is the most commonly used traction type tube for palliation of esophagogastric carcinoma. The technique of insertion (Fig. 21) requires both esophagoscopy and a laparotomy with a gastrotomy incision, usually performed under general anesthesia. If possible, a leaded string is swallowed preoperatively to allow accurate passage of dilators and the tube introducer through the tumor. Esophagoscopy then localizes

---

*Manufactured by Ambleletin, Ltd., P.O. Box 1, Tetbury Glos. GL8 8TL

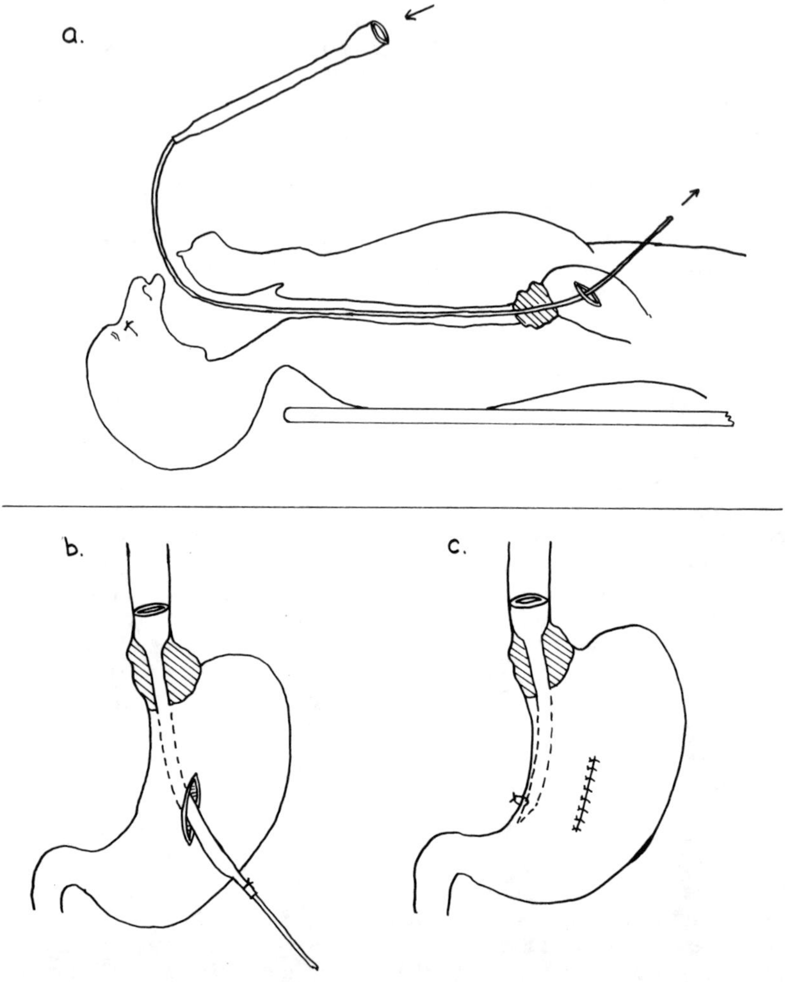

Figure 21: Insertion of traction type (Celestin) intraluminal tube to palliate dysphagia.

accurately the level of the proximal part of the obstruction, dilators are passed progressively to assure easy passage of the tube. A small laparotomy just large enough to expose the anterior stomach is made. A small gastrotomy is made in the midportion of the stomach drawing out the string through the gastrotomy. The string is attached to the tube introducer at the mouth and the introducer is pulled through the esophagus and out the gastrotomy. If no string has been passed, the introducer is passed blindly through the tumor into the stomach. The Celestin tube is then pulled through the lesion using the introducer until the proximal flange of the tube is felt to lodge in the proximal portion of the obstructing tumor. The position of the proximal flange is then checked by repeat esophagoscopy. When the proper position is assured, the end of the tube is cut diagonally across with the open end toward the lumen of the stomach and sutured to the inside wall of the less curvature of the stomach with a horizontal mattress suture of O-polypropylene through full thickness stomach wall and tied without tension outside the stomach.

Postoperatively the head of the patient's bed is maintained elevated at 30° to prevent reflux and aspiration. The diet is advanced to a blenderized diet as tolerated. Some patients are able to resume a relatively normal diet as long as they chew their food thoroughly before swallowing. Carbonated beverages after meals seem to help in keeping the tubes open.

There are a number of reports emphasizing the safety of the Celestin tube and other traction type tubes (135-138); however, in most series reporting a large experience with traction type prosthetic tubes, there is a significant incidence of mortality and morbidity associated with their use. Saunders (139) reported the use of Celestin tube palliation of esophageal carcinoma in 116 patients. There was a 30% operative mortality and 53% three-month mortality. Complications in these patients were common with bronchopneumonia occurring in 28% of patients, wound infection in 20%, esophageal perforation in 10%, empyema in 7%, displaced tube in 3%, and gastric fistula in 1. 7%. Angorn (146) reported similar results with a 33% operative mortality, esophageal leak in 10%, and hemorrhage from the esophagus or stomach in 6%. He reported successful intubation in 71% of upper esophageal tumors but in only 47% of lower esophageal tumors. In his hands, resection was safer than intubation. In Pringles series of 34 patients (95), only 16 of 34 (47%) left the hospital with satisfactory swallowing. In long-term survivals of Celestin tube placement, there is concern about the possible dissolution of the tube as has been reported by Rao (140). These dismal results are not difficult to understand when one considers that most of these patients are poorly nourished, have far advanced metastatic disease, but are desperate for the ability to swallow. To subject such patients to general anesthesia, a laparotomy, and then open gastroesophageal reflux postoperatively is a large insult.

Recognizing this high incidence of complications with the traction type tubes, a resurgence of interest has developed in the use of pulsion type tubes such as the Souttar tube or the newer and larger Proctor-Livingstone* tube. The technique for insertion of this latter tube (Fig. 22) is to visualize the tumor with a large Negus esophagoscope and dilate the lumen through the tumor to a 38 French gauge. A smaller bougie is left across the tumor and the prosthetic is then pushed into place with the esophagoscope and a special pusher. The use of a preoperatively

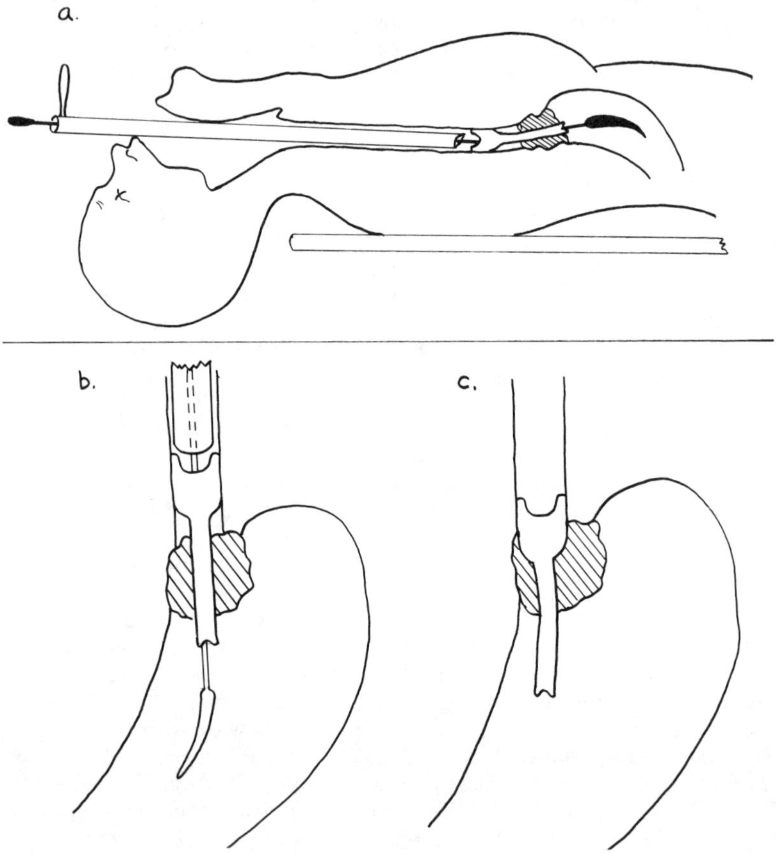

Figure 22: Insertion of pulsion type (Proctor-Livingstone) tube.

*Manufactured by Latex Products, P.O. Box 5626, Johannesburg 2000, South Africa.

swallowed string through the lumen of the esophagus aids in safe passage of the dilators and the tube through the tumor. In high tumors the tube is cut so that the distal end of the tube lies beyond the tumor but above the esophagogastric junction, which helps in preventing reflux. In lower tumors the end must necessarily lie in the stomach. Atkinson (141) has described a technique whereby a pulsion type tube can be inserted using a fiberoptic endoscope. The postoperative care is similar to that after Celestin tube insertion.

Generally the results after intubation with a pulsion type tube are superior to those with a traction type tube, chiefly in the reduction of operative mortality by avoiding a laparotomy and gastrotomy, but there is more frequent migration with the pulsion tubes since they are not suture fixed to the stomach as are the traction tubes. Zimmerman (93) reported on 50 patients who had Souttar tubes placed for esophageal cancer. There was only one operative death (2° to perforation), but there were 22 patients in which the tube migrated (most of these were distal migrations after radiation therapy). All of these tubes either remained in the stomach or passed distally without difficulty. Palmer (142) described a new pulsion tube used in 62 patients without an operative death and with very few complications. Hegarty (143) used the Proctor-Livingstone tube in 181 patients with a 16% operative mortality rate, which was one-half the mortality rate he had previously noted with the Celestin tube. He noted 13 of 181 (7.2%) proximal migrations of the tube, all of which were easily reinserted and two of 181 (1.1%) distal migrations. Ammann (97) compared 30 patients with Souttar tube placement to 29 patients with Mousseau-Barbin tube placement and found the differences between the tubes attributable to the higher mortality associated with the insertion of the traction type tube.

Our practice is to use a traction type tube (Celestin tube preferentially) when the decision for use of a prosthetic tube is made at exploratory staging laparotomy, because there is a lesser tendency for migration of the tube if it can be anchored to the stomach wall and the risk of laparotomy has already been committed. When the need for prosthetic intubation of the esophagus can be determined before laparotomy (such as the patient with advanced systemic metastases and esophageal obstruction) we prefer a pulsion type tube (our choice is the Proctor-Livingstone tube or a self-made tube of heavy rubber), avoiding the risk of laparotomy but accepting a greater risk of tube migration.

The use of prosthetic tubes to bridge malignant esophago-respiratory fistulae has proven very valuable and generally superior to any other form of palliation of this grave condition.

Lolley (144) reported 46 patients treated for this condition by five treatment modalities. Seven patients were treated with supportive therapy alone with an average survival of six days and none left the hospital. Ten patients were treated with gastrostomy and tracheostomy with an average survival of two and one-half weeks, only two of eight obtaining palliation and only one patient left the hospital. Four patients were treated with diversion and exclusion procedures with an average survival of three and one-half weeks, three were not palliated and only one left the hospital. Prosthetic endoesophageal intubation was used on 20 patients with an average survival of five months, 16 patients left the hospital with fair to good palliation and there were only two operative deaths. The last group was a very select group of five patients with very favorable tumors who underwent colon bypass and occasional resection. Four of five had good palliation with an average survival of 18 months and there was one long-term survival after resection. Hegarty (145) found the use of the Proctor-Livingstone tube superior to the Celestin tube in palliation of esophagorespiratory fistulae. He was able to intubate all patients, but with a 64.3% mortality using Celestin tubes compared to 25% mortality with Proctor-Livingstone tube. There was good palliation in the survivors.

Radiation

Radiation of carcinoma of the distal esophagus and esophagogastric junction for palliation is generally of limited usefulness. To achieve relief of the obstruction usually requires high dose radiation between 4000 to 6000 r over four to six weeks of treatments and often requires repeated dilatations to achieve an open lumen in the esophagus, both of which are generally miserable experiences to the patient. Relief of the dysphagia after radiation is usually delayed for several weeks. After a period of several months of relief, the dysphagia often recurs either from recurrent carcinoma or from fibrous stricture, and then further dilatations and often a prosthetic tube are required to maintain swallowing. In Friedman's series of patients undergoing radiation therapy for carcinoma of the esophagus (112), 90% of the patients had some degree of resultant stenosis with recurrent dysphagia in 22%. In Pearson's series (113), 27% of his patients required dilatation postradiation to maintain swallowing and only 41% returned to a normal diet. For all these reasons, we generally limit palliative radiation for use in some patients with widespread metastases detected preoperatively or some patients with unresectable primary lesions and gross liver or peritoneal metastases when nonresectional palliation for a limited time period is desired. Most of these situations are more expediently handled by prosthetic intubation, but when intubation fails radiation may be desirable.

Simple Resection

Simple resection of carcinoma of the esophagus, particularly the distal esophagus and cardia with reconstruction by esophagogastrostomy, has proven to be a valuable form of palliation in appropriate patients. Such a resection removes the obstructing lesion including the gross tumor margins and immediately adjacent tumor bearing nodes if possible. Lasting palliation of dysphagia is rapidly achieved; there is relatively little morbidity and mortality to the procedure; and excellent swallowing is generally provided. Angorn (146) randomized 95 patients with incurable carcinoma of the esophagus to resection versus Celestin tube intubation for palliation of dysphagia. There was a significantly better response to resection versus intubation with 10% versus 44% operative mortality, 80% versus 47% of patients discharged swallowing, and 40% versus 2% one-year survival. Hankins (147) performed palliative resection in 45 of 46 patients with middle and lower esophageal carcinomas with 20% operative mortality and excellent palliation. We generally perform a palliative resection when the patient is a suitable candidate for surgery; the tumor is resectable but incurable and yet there are not widespread metastases denoting a very limited survival time.

Palliative Bypass

Palliative bypass of the obstructing carcinomas using a colon interposition or gastric bypass has been advocated by many. In each instance the organ for bypass has generally been brought up to the cervical esophagus for anastomosis by either a subcutaneous or a substernal route, thereby avoiding a thoracotomy and an intrathoracic anastomosis. Ong (148) has advocated a return to the Kirschner operation where the stomach is brought up subcutaneously to anastomose to the cervical esophagus, a feat we have found to be difficult possibly because of the difference in relative length of the esophagus in American patients as opposed to the Japanese, which has recently been demonstrated by Goldsmith (149). Orringer (150) and Akiyama (151) prefer substernal gastric bypass of the thoracic esophagus for palliation of esophageal carcinoma. For carcinomas of the esophagogastric junction, however, total mobilization of stomach for use as a bypass to the cervical esophagus is usually impossible because of tumor invasion of the proximal stomach. We, therefore, prefer a substernal colon interposition as a palliative bypass of an unresectable lesion of the esophagogastric junction when the patient appears capable of tolerating the procedure and there are few or no metastases to limit survival.

The general preoperative preparation for colon interposition to bypass a carcinoma of the esophagus or cardia is carried out as described later for radical esophagogastrectomy including hyperalimentation, pulmonary hygiene, and monitoring. As has been urged by Wilkins (152), we prefer to carry out a thorough preoperative examination of the colon with a barium enema and angiography to determine the presence of any colon pathology, especially diverticulosis, and to examine the actual blood supply of the colon in order to be able to select that portion of the colon for the bypass that is free of pathology and has adequate blood supply. The blood supply to the right colon is less predictable than that to the left and transverse colon; however, in these older patients with carcinoma, any of the vessels may be involved by atherosclerotic disease, particularly the inferior mesenteric artery. Combined mechanical and oral antibiotic preparation of the colon is done as outlined by Nichols (Table 3) (153).

A long, midline abdominal incision is made; or if the indication for the colon interposition is determined at the exploratory laparotomy prior to a planned esophageal resection, that incision is extended downward in the midline to provide full exposure of the abdomen. Both the right and the left colon are mobilized fully

Table 3 Neomycin-Erythromycin Base Colon Preparation

Day 1:	Low residue diet Bisacodyl, one capsule orally at 6 pm	
Day 2:	Continue low residue diet Magnesium sulfate 30 ml 50% solution (15 g) orally at 10 am, 2 pm, and 6 pm Saline enemas in evening until return clear	
Day 3:	Clear liquid diet; supplemental IV fluids as needed Magnesium sulfate, in dose above, at 10 am and 2 pm No enemas	
	Neomycin 1 g	p.o. at 1 pm
	Erythromycin base 1 g	2 pm and 11 pm
Day 4:	Operation scheduled at 8 am	

Nichols et al. (153)

from their lateral reflections. Particular care must be exercised at the splenic flexure to avoid injury to the spleen. The greater omentum is detached from the transverse colon leaving its attachment to the greater curvature of the stomach. Using the information of the preoperative angiogram and/or transillumination of the mesentery of the colon, the vascularity of the colon is carefully analysed to determine which part is appropriate to create a long pedicle which will reach to the neck. The marginal artery of Drummond between the middle colic artery and the left colic artery is a much more reliable vascular arch than is the marginal artery communication between the right or middle colic artery and the ileocolic artery. For this reason, our preference is to use the left transverse and descending colon for the bypass based either on the middle colic artery or on the left colic artery (Fig. 23A). This segment of colon is also preferable over the ascending colon because its diameter more nearly approaches that of the esophagus and allows passage

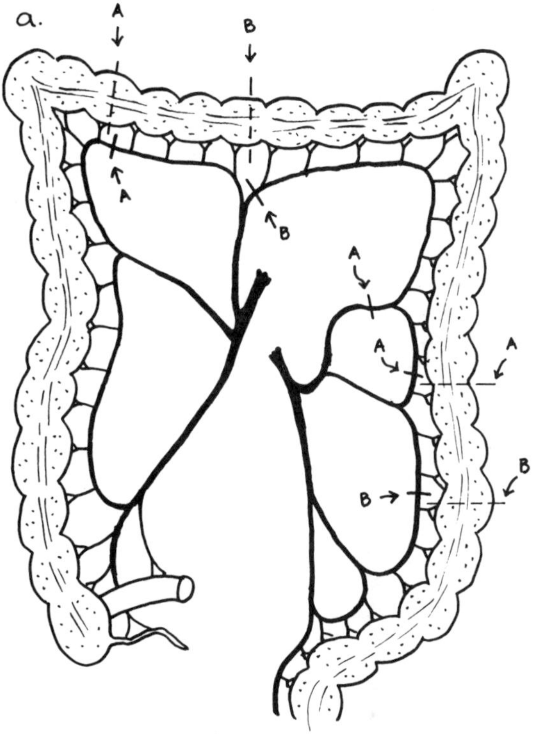

Figure 23A: Use of the left transverse and descending colon for esophageal interposition. Resection when the colon is based on the middle colic artery.

through the thoracic inlet into the neck more easily. Since the segmental peristalsis of the colon allows the colon to be used in either an isoperistaltic or retroperistaltic direction, either artery is acceptable. The mesentery of the chosen section of colon is divided sharply, very close to the level of the vascular arcade. If the pedicle is to be based on the left colic artery, the middle colic artery is temporarily occluded with a soft sponge Brown clamp to assure the viability of the proposed pedicle; then the vessel is divided. If the pedicle will be based on the middle colic artery, the left colic artery is occluded in a similar fashion. Finally the colon is divided at a point several centimeters longer than the measured distance to the cervical esophagus to assure enough length. The other end is also divided and the remaining intestinal segments are reattached by an end-to-end two-layered inverting anastomosis and the mesentery is re-approximated.

Meanwhile, the cervical incision is made parallel to the anterior border of the left sternomastoid muscle. This muscle and the carotid sheath are reflected laterally and the esophagus is dissected free for several centimeters below the cricopharyngeus muscle with care to avoid injury to the recurrent laryngeal nerves.

The retrosternal tunnel is then created by blunt dissection from above and below avoiding entrance into the pleura. This is enlarged until the entire hand and forearm can pass easily through this tunnel to the neck. If the thoracic inlet is particularly tight, a portion of the manubrium and left clavicle may be removed for more room.

The colon pedicle is then passed behind the stomach, through the gastrohepatic ligament, and then through the tunnel to the neck, taking great care not to twist the colon on itself and not to compress its venous drainage (Fig. 23B). The most proximal end of the colon, which has been closed with a two-layer inverting closure, is attached by several sutures to the prevertebral fascia a few centimeters above the proposed esophagocolic anastomosis. The esophagus is divided five to six cm below the cricopharyngeus and the distal end closed in two layers. The proximal end of the esophagus is then anastomosed to the side of the colon with a two-layered anastomosis of interrupted sutures. We use 4-0 Dexon or Vicryl for the inner layer and 3-0 permanent sutures for the outer layer. A suction catheter is passed through the nose and esophagus into the colon for post-operative decompression. The distal end of the colon is then anastomosed end-to-side to the anterior wall of the stomach in its midportion.

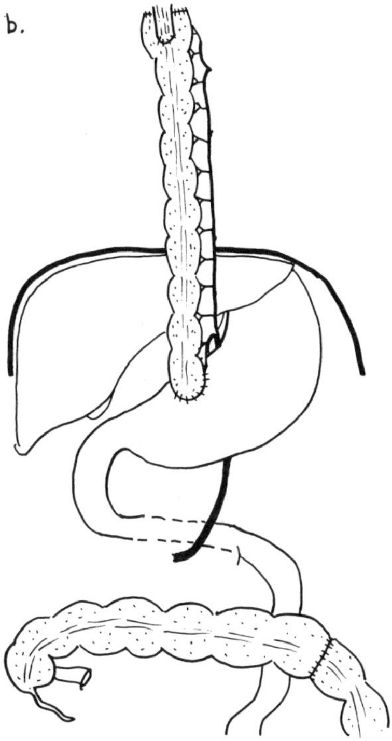

Figure 23B: Use of the left transverse and descending colon for esophageal interposition. Resection when the colon is based on the left colic artery. Colon pedicle passes behind the stomach and through the lesser omentum to the retrosternal space.

If the right ascending colon is to be used, the technical steps are similar (Fig. 24). The pedicle is based on the right colic artery, and the cecum and distal ileum are passed through the retrosternal tunnel into the neck. The cecum is tacked to the prevertebral fascia and the anastomosis is made between the esophagus and cecum. The ileum can then be brought through the incision for decompression and closed at a later date.

Postoperatively, the patient is not allowed to swallow liquids until the ileus has resolved. Only clear liquids are then allowed until a barium swallow is obtained on the seventh to tenth postoperative day. If the anastomoses are intact the diet is rapidly advanced as tolerated. If a small leak is present (rare in the cologastric anastomosis but not uncommon in the cervical anastomosis) food is withheld for another ten days until a repeat barium swallow demonstrates healing of the fistula.

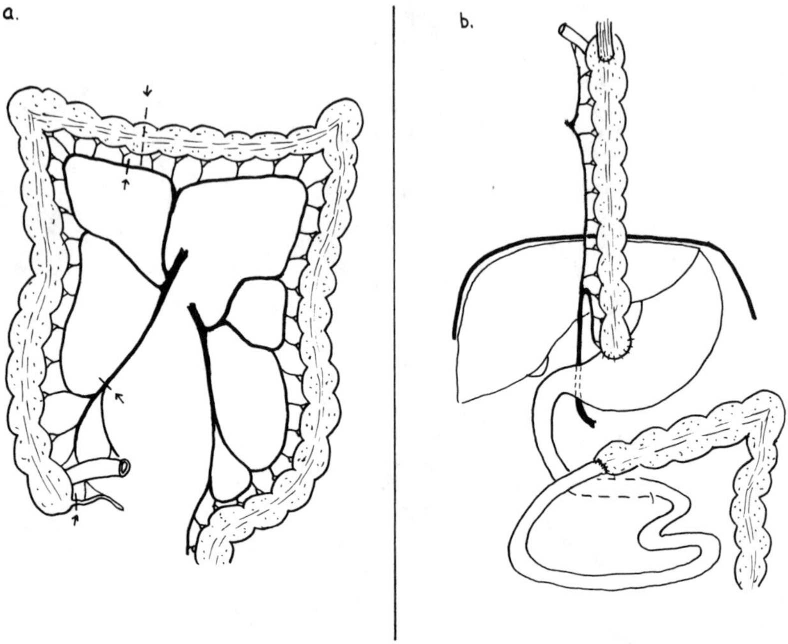

Figure 24: Use of the ascending and right transverse colon for esophageal interposition.

Fortunately leaks of the esophagocolic anastomosis in the neck almost invariably heal unless there is total disruption of the suture line.

Mullen (154) reported the results in 43 patients plus a general review of 15 other authors, noting an overall mortality rate for substernal colon interposition of 11.9%. Bowel necrosis was observed in 8%, proximal anastomotic leak in 20 to 30%, and later stricture in 20%. Two cases of duodenal obstruction occurred when the vascular pedicle of the colon was left anterior to the stomach. Belsey (155) reported 105 cases of reconstruction of the esophagus with left colon with a 4.8% mortality. He noted two cases of colon necrosis secondary to venous obstruction and infarction, two cases of cervical leaks, three pleural infections, and two wound infections; Petrov (156) reported 100 patients who had retrosternal colon interposition with 7% mortality and 9% additional patients with partial or complete colon necrosis. In Wilkins' series of 30 retrosternal colon interpositions, he had only one death.

Chemotherapy

Chemotherapy of gastroesophageal cancer has, until recently, been rather unrewarding. The drugs and/or drug combinations available to treat such tumors have not been very effective in most patients. In addition, the type of patient usually referred to the chemotherapist was in such poor physical condition or had such widespread disease that the chances of success were remote, even if effective chemotherapy regimens had been available. Finally, whatever tumor shrinkage might have resulted from treatment was difficult or impossible to evaluate, as the bulk of measurable disease was hidden in the abdomen. Despite this gloomy background, chemotherapy continues to be the only hope for improved survival or quality of life once surgery and radiation have failed, and that is the case in the majority of patients. We will, therefore, give a brief overview of the drugs and drug regimens which are available to treat such individuals.

The most active single agent in the treatment of gut adenocarcinomas is 5-Fluorouracil (157). About 15 to 20% of patients show some type of response to this drug, which lasts about four to five months. While occasional responses may be dramatic in nature, in most instances, complete disappearance of the tumor does not occur and survival is not significantly lengthened. Combinations of 5-Fluorouracil with Adriamycin, or with Adriamycin plus Mitomycin-C may, however, give response rates as high as 43% in advanced gastric cancer and, in addition, improve survival over that seen with 5-Fluorouracil alone (158, 159). We have been using the combination of 5-Fluorouracil, Adriamycin, and Mitomycin-C for the past several years in patients with advanced pancreatic or gastric adenocarcinoma and found it easy to deliver and well tolerated. Median survival in the patients so treated is about six months. Because all patients had only intra-abdominal disease, however, response rates have been impossible to quantify, even with the CT scan.

There is less experience to draw from in the chemotherapy of squamous carcinoma of the esophagus. Such tumors are less common than gut adenocarcinomas, and the percentage of the former referred to the chemotherapist is smaller than the percentage of the latter. As a result, the drug regimens most commonly employed in esophageal cancer have been those in use for squamous cancer of the lung or head and neck. The most effective single agents in the former disease are Cytoxan, Adriamycin, Methotrexate, and CCNU, with response rates ranging from 15 to 25% and a median duration of response of two to three months (160). Various combinations of these agents, such as MACC (Methotrexate, Adriamycin, Cytoxan, CCNU) or CAMP

(Cytoxan, Adriamycin, Methotrexate, Procarbazine), are claimed to increase the response rate to 40 to 50% (161,162). We, however, have not been able to duplicate this experience and our response rates with these combinations have been closer to 20%.

Single agents which are reasonably effective in squamous head and neck cancer include Methotrexate, Bleomycin, Hydroxyurea, Cytoxan, Vinblastine, Adriamycin, and more recently, Cis-Platinum (163,164). Reported response rates with these agents range from 25 to 40%; however, the median duration of such responses is only two months (163). Two promising combinations in head and neck cancer are Bleomycin plus Cis-Platinum and Methotrexate, Bleomycin plus Cis-Platinum (165, 166). Response rates with these combinations range from 50 to 80% (165-167); however, few of the patients in these studies had disease which had recurred in a radiation port. Our experience in both head and neck cancer, as well as that of the esophagus, is that tumor recurrence in a previously radiated field is unlikely to respond to any of the single agents or drug combinations seen above. Because of that, we have now begun to use a five drug combination which employs Cytoxan, Adriamycin, CCNU, Vincristine, and Cis-Platinum (168), and are beginning to see responses in lung and recurrent (postradiation) head and neck cancer where we never saw them before. A few patients with recurrent squamous esophageal cancer have also been treated with encouraging early results.

Selective Therapy Scheme

The selective therapy scheme (Table 2) has been devised based on our interpretation of the treatment alternatives discussed above. Unless the patient has obvious widespread metastases, has invasion of the respiratory tract, or is medically inoperable because of other diseases, he is prepared for surgery which is immediately preceded by an exploratory laparotomy. The findings at laparotomy, as particularly regards resectability of the primary carcinoma and the presence or absence of metastases outside the resection margins, determine the further course of therapy as radical resection, radiation, palliative resection, palliative bypass, or palliative intubation. A more elaborate discussion of these treatment alternatives will be discussed later under the discussion of surgical resection.

SURGICAL RESECTION OF CARCINOMA OF THE ESOPHAGOGASTRIC JUNCTION

Preoperative Considerations

General

Generally, after the patient has undergone barium swallow, esophagoscopy, and bronchoscopy (if indicated) to confirm the diagnosis of carcinoma of the distal esophagus or esophagogastric junction, selection of the appropriate form of therapy is made. Unless there is a specific contraindication, our policy has been to prepare all patients with esophagogastric cancer for exploratory laparotomy and esophagogastrectomy as a single stage procedure. Specific contraindications to this usual route of therapy include: (1) tracheal or bronchial involvement as demonstrated by bronchoscopy (unusual in carcinoma of the distal esophagus or esophagogastric junction); (2) pulmonary metastases as noted on routine preoperative chest X-ray (The common sites of distal metastases are liver, lung, adrenals, and kidneys. Of these only the lung metastases can be accurately and practically determined prior to laparotomy.); (3) prohibitive cardiac or pulmonary conditions that cannot be improved prior to surgery (severe congestive heart failure and severe chronic obstructive lung disease); (4) involvement of cervical or upper mediastinal lymph nodes as demonstrated by a biopsy positive supraclavicular node or documented left recurrent nerve palsy (Routine mediastinoscopy is not advocated in lower esophageal carcinoma.) (103, 104); (5) general inanition noncorrected by hyperalimentation and general care (The presumption is made that this severe debility is from metastases rather than starvation, so great care must be exercised in making this judgment.).

Patients who are so selected not to undergo exploration and resection must be considered for palliation of their dysphagia by radiation or esophageal intubation. Pulsion intubation is generally preferred as described previously. For those patients headed for exploratory laparotomy, and probably resection, very careful preparations must be made to minimize the morbidity and mortality of the procedure.

Nutrition and Hydration

Nutrition and hydration are affected because of the associated dysphagia in most patients with esophagogastric carcinoma. These patients will be suffering from malnutrition and dehydration of some degree. The degree of malnutrition (generally measured as weight loss) is related to the severity of the dysphagia and not necessarily to the extent of carcinoma spread. This degree of malnutrition has been correlated to the ability to withstand a major operative procedure. Overall complication rates (169, 170) and problems of wound healing (171) have been shown to be markedly increased in malnourished patients and also to be improved by pre- and postoperative hyperalimentation in patients with esophageal carcinoma. Nonspecific cellular and humoral immune response is markedly compromised in malnourished patients with esophageal carcinoma, and reversal of the negative-nitrogen balance by hyperalimentation improves this immune response (172), a finding that may bear directly on the high susceptibility of these patients to postoperative wound and pulmonary infection complications.

For these reasons, our general policy is to administer pre- and postoperative intravenous hyperalimentation to any patient with greater than 15% weight loss. With increasing experience we have found intravenous hyperalimentation via a carefully placed and meticulously cared for central venous catheter to be a much more reliable method of administering calories, fluid, and vitamins preoperatively in the patient with severe dysphagia and fraught now with less complications than the administration of enteral calories by nasogastric tube, gastrostomy, or ileostomy. Occasionally in the patient with little or only mild dysphagia, oral administration of calorie-rich fluids with vitamins is used, but our experience suggests that this is successful only occasionally. We aim for the administration of 50 to 60 kcal/kg and 0.3 to 0.4 gm/kg of nitrogen per day plus appropriate minerals and vitamins for seven to ten days preoperatively and until a satisfactory diet is being swallowed postoperatively (usually another seven to ten days). The continuation of this steady dose of hyperalimentation throughout the operative procedure is a basic principle in intravenous hyperalimentation. We do not routinely measure nitrogen balance since previous studies have shown that this level of hyperalimentation will generally return the patient to positive nitrogen balance and hold him there through the procedure (171). Gastrostomy for alimentation prior to surgery is to be particularly avoided because of its interference in the use of the stomach as an esophageal replacement later. Standard jejunostomy is advocated by some, but we have found that patients generally tolerate jejunostomy feedings poorly with long delays in achieving good alimentation without excess diarrhea by this route. The use of elemental diets via a needle catheter jejunostomy as advocated by Hoover (173) may be helpful in enteral feedings particularly postoperatively.

Contrary to a long-held belief, patients with malignant esophageal obstruction and weight loss are not hypovolemic and do not require preoperative transfusions of blood or plasma (174). Extravascular fluid, however, is often reduced so we generally assure that the patient is receiving adequate fluid volume (either orally or parenterally) for several days prior to surgery meaning 40 to 50 cc/kg/day.

Pulmonary Hygiene

Aggressive pulmonary hygiene both pre- and postoperatively is extremely important for several reasons. Patients with esophagogastric carcinoma frequently have preexisting chronic obstructive pulmonary disease which if neglected will provide major problems in the postoperative period. Patients with any degree of esophageal obstruction and particularly severe malignant obstruction usually have some degree of aspiration pneumonitis. The contemplated resection involves both an upper abdominal and a thoracic incision, both of which individually and in combination are well-known to be associated with postoperative pulmonary problems. Accordingly we recommend: (1) routine preoperative pulmonary function tests and arterial blood gas determinations; (2) routine sputum culture with treatment of any pathogenic organisms with a seven to ten day course of the appropriate antibiotics; (3) no smoking for at least seven days preoperatively; (4) vigorous exercises by trained technicians or nurses in postural drainage, deep breathing, and coughing for two to three days preoperatively, routinely and for longer as necessary in patients with preexisting lung disease or active pneumonitis or bronchitis; (5) vigorous treatment of any bronchospastic element of chronic lung disease. The use of aminophylline is particularly recommended since this drug can be given orally or parenterally and blood levels can be monitored. Obviously these measures must also be carried into the postoperative period.

Preparations for Possible Colon Interposition

Preparations for a possible colon interposition are made in all operations involving resection of the gastroesophageal junction should this be necessary at the time of surgery. First, a consideration of the potential vascularity of the colon is made. If there is evidence of generalized vascular disease or specifically aortoiliac vascular disease, we recommend angiography to demonstrate the vascular anatomy of the colon preoperatively to determine which portion of the colon is best suited for transplantation into the thorax. Second, we routinely do a colon prep as recommended by Nichols (153) (Table 3).

Intraoperative Monitoring

Intraoperative monitoring is being used to an ever-increasing degree during the radical resection of a carcinoma of the esophagogastric junction, due to the significant physiological insult to the patient, particularly any patient with compromised cardiac or pulmonary function. The fluid shifts from intra- to extravascular spaces are as large as that seen in abdominal aortic procedures and often go unappreciated. In addition, arterial oxygenation may be diminished by compromised lungs. For these reasons, we have employed detailed monitoring to an ever-increasing degree. Presently we consider the minimal necessary monitoring during the operation and early postoperative period to consist of: (1) continuous EKG and arterial blood pressure; (2) hourly central venous pressure measurements; (3) hourly recording of fluid intake and output with an indwelling urinary catheter in place; (4) continuous positive-pressure respiration by a mechanical respirator for 12 to 24 hours minimum; (5) frequent measurement of arterial blood gases and pH. In addition, whenever the patient has pre-existing cardiac disease of significant extent, or in any situation in which the fluid volume or cardiac function is unclear from the previous methods, we readily employ a balloon tipped pulmonary artery catheter to measure pulmonary artery wedge pressure and cardiac output according to the thermodilution technique (Swam-Ganz^{R} Flow-Directed Thermodilution Catheter, Model 93A-131-7F*). Using these careful monitoring techniques, we now rarely have major difficulty with the cardiovascular system in the operative or postoperative period, and pulmonary problems are decreased by accurate fluid management.

Intraoperative Care

Exploratory Laparotomy

Exploratory laparotomy has provided the most accurate and direct method of staging and determining the appropriate management of carcinoma of the distal esophagus and esophagogastric junction. The predominant spread from the primary site of malignancy is first by direct lateral extension of growth through the esophageal wall and by submucosal spread within the esophagus and stomach; second, by metastases to the regional nodes of the lesser curvature of the stomach, eventually to the celiac

---

*Edwards Laboratories, Inc.

axis, the nodes in splenic hilum, along the superior border of the pancreas, and the paraesophageal nodes leading to the nodes of the subcarinal and perihilar region; and third, by distant metastatic spread to the liver, adrenals, kidneys, general peritoneal cavity, and lung. As has been previously discussed, noninvasive techniques have been of little help and are often misleading in determining the extent of this spread. In our experience, exploratory laparotomy has provided the most accurate and direct method of staging and determining the appropriate management of carcinomas in this location. As is readily apparent in the algorithm of selective therapy (Table 2), the exploratory laparotomy forms the focal point from which most management decisions are made.

It has been our practice to perform the exploratory laparotomy after the patient has undergone all of the preoperative preparations that have been detailed in the previous section and immediately prior to a planned resection of the carcinoma to be carried out under the same anesthetic, depending on the results of the exploratory laparotomy. All surgical alternatives based on the laparotomy findings can immediately be determined and applied, and this practice allows one to maximize the safety of both the laparotomy and the more extensive resection procedure.

The position of the patient and the incision for the laparotomy are determined by the approach selected for the definitive resection. If a left thoracoabdominal incision is planned for the resection, the patient is placed in a standard right lateral position, but with the pelvis tilted back toward the supine approximately 45°, and the incision is made from the midline in the midepigastrium to the costal margin at the rib or interspace where the thoracic portion of the incision is planned (usually the seventh rib). If the Lewis approach with a separate abdominal incision and a right thoracotomy is planned for the definitive resection, a midline abdominal incision from the xyphoid to the umbilicus is made.

Through either of these incisions a thorough exploration of the abdomen is made. Particular attention is directed to three major concerns: (1) Is there metastatic spread of carcinoma outside of the resection margins of a radical resection? Specific note should be made of the presence or absence of liver metastases, palpable metastases in adrenals or kidneys, metastases in lymph nodes of the porta hepatis or along the aorta below the pancreas, and peritoneal seeding of carcinoma. If there are metastases outside of the margins of a radical resection, such a resection should not be undertaken; however, a simple palliative resection may be indicated for relief of dysphagia. Simple enlargement of lymph nodes can be misleading so all suspected metastases must be confirmed by frozen section pathology. Liver metastases are usually obvious, but should always be confirmed by biopsy with frozen sections at the time if there is a question or if needle biopsy is necessary to verify a mass deep in the liver. There should be no question about the presence or absence of metastases at the end of the exploratory laparotomy. The presence of metastatic nodes at the celiac axis does not in itself preclude an attempt at resection even if these nodes initially feel "fixed." There have been reports of long-term survival after resection of esophagogastric carcinoma with involvement of the celiac nodes (175). Only if further dissection reveals that the involved nodes at the celiac axis are truly unresectable because of invasion into the hepatic artery branch of the celiac axis or into the wall of the aorta should the dissection be abandoned; (2) Is there evidence of unresectability of the primary lesion at the esophagogastric junction? Carcinomas higher in the esophagus are generally unassessable from a laparotomy incision, but lesions at the esophagogastric junction can usually be fairly-well evaluated. Unresectability is based on direct extension of the lesion into surrounding unresectable structures, especially the aorta, the vertebral bodies, or extensively into the liver or into the retroperitoneum involving directly the left adrenal and/or kidney. The adventitia of the aorta, the diaphragm at the hiatus, or minor direct invasion of the left lobe of the liver or of easily resectable retroperitoneal tissue does not preclude en bloc resection. Once resectability is determined to be feasible from the abdominal side of the diaphragm, a final decision of resectability must be determined later from the thoracic approach; (3) What is the extent of the primary tumor involvement of the stomach and the extent of node metastases within the margins of resection? The decision of how radical an abdominal resection is to be undertaken will be based on this determination.

The results of the exploratory laparotomy provide the information necessary to immediately decide what appropriate further operative therapy should be undertaken or what general plan of palliative therapy should be planned. These laparotomy findings and the subsequent routes of therapy can be divided into four major categories as outlined on the treatment algorithm (Table 2).

Unresectable Metastases with a Resectable Primary Carcinoma: Radical resection of this lesion is unwarranted since all of the tumor cannot be removed, and such a resection does not prolong life but does subject the patient to the morbidity and mortality of such a major resection. Generally the survival in this circumstance will be short, rarely greater than six months; therefore, the treatment plan should be aimed at maximum palliation with the least morbidity and mortality, and with the aim toward minimal time in the hospital.

If there has been significant dysphagia prior to surgery, attention is directed to rapid palliation of that dysphagia. When the resectable primary is small, we advise a simple resection of the primary with margins adequate to prevent rapid recurrence and simple esophagogastrostomy with a fundal wrap of the anastomosis to prevent reflux. Occasionally this may be possible through a laparotomy incision, but it usually requires that the thoracotomy be made to provide adequate exposure. Transection of the costal margin is not necessary for such a limited resection. Obviously, this decision to do a limited resection for palliation must be based on the surgeon's confidence and experience in doing esophagogastric anastomoses without a significant incidence of anastomotic leak or other major complications. When the resectable primary is large and would require an extensive resection, we advise an attempt at intubation of the esophagus, generally with a traction type tube such as the Celestin tube, with guidance from both an esophagoscope above and a gastrotomy below to assure the safe placement of the tube across the lesion. Limited resection is used if intubation is found to be impossible or if a perforation from the intubation attempt is noted at the time. Generally, we reserve radiation for palliation of the primary in this circumstance only if in our judgment resection is inadvisable and intubation is technically impossible, since radiation requires several weeks to achieve relief of the obstruction and carries its own morbidity as previously discussed.

If there has been no significant dysphagia prior to surgery then in the presence of unresectable metastases resection of the primary lesion is not advised. The later intubation of the esophagus when dysphagia becomes a significant problem is indicated. Generally we prefer a pulsion type tube, such as the Proctor-Livingstone tube in this circumstance, because this tube requires less of an operative procedure, less hospitalization time, and appears to carry less overall morbidity and mortality than a traction type tube requiring a separate laparotomy for its placement.

Prophylactic radiation to a primary esophageal carcinoma in the presence of unresectable metastases but without dysphagia is advocated by some radiation therapists, but its efficacy in preventing the subsequent development of significant dysphagia prior to death from metastatic carcinoma has not been demonstrated. Radiation may be chosen later as an alternative to intubation of the esophagus when dysphagia does occur.

Unresectable Metastases with an Unresectable Primary Carcinoma: In this circumstance, the primary goal of therapy, again, is palliation of dysphagia which is invariably a significant problem in these large tumors. Again, survival is rarely more than a few months, so the overall circumstance does not warrant the morbidity and mortality of a major operative procedure such as colon interposition or other extraanatomic bypass. Esophageal intubation is generally the treatment of choice. Since these circumstances are noted at the exploratory laparotomy, a traction type tube is generally employed. On rare occasions, when the fundus of the stomach is not involved by carcinoma, a limited bypass such as described by Johnson and Claggett (176) (Fig. 25) may be employed for palliation in this circumstance. Radiation may also be used by the usual large size of these tumors and the time necessary for treatment generally preclude its usefulness.

Unresectable Primary Carcinoma Without Metastases or with Metastases Limited to Nodes Adjacent to the Primary Carcinoma: This group of patients have a more favorable prognosis than the previous two groups of patients. Their immediate survival and comfort are primarily threatened by starvation from esophageal obstruction. With adequate palliation of their dysphagia, death from metastases generally is delayed for many months and occasionally several years. With radical radiation therapy to the primary lesion, occasional five-year survivals

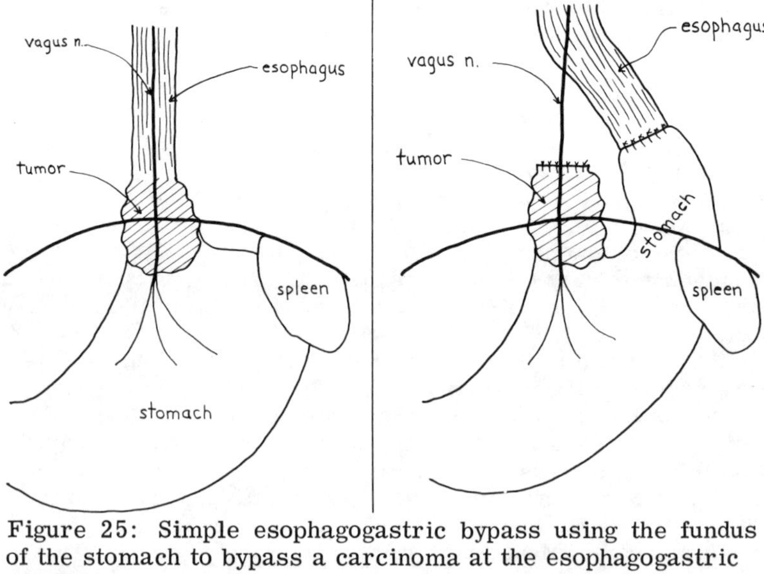

Figure 25: Simple esophagogastric bypass using the fundus of the stomach to bypass a carcinoma at the esophagogastric junction.

are reported (113, 116,118). Accordingly, we are generally aggressive in our approach to these lesions.

If the dysphagia has been very significant (as is the usual case), a substernal colon interposition between the cervical esophagus and the stomach is created, then after recovery from the surgery (usually 10 to 14 days), the patient is referred to the radiation therapists for radical radiation of the primary carcinoma according to the general guidelines laid down by Pearson (113). The reasons for preferring a substernal colon bypass in this situation are several: (1) thoracotomy is not necessary and patients generally tolerate this surgery very well; (2) although there are anastomoses involved, all are outside of the thorax so that the consequences of an occasional anastomotic leak (almost exclusively limited to the cervical anastomosis) are minimal; and (3) the colon bypass and all anastomoses are well away from the primary carcinoma, so there is little likelihood of their being involved by spread of the carcinoma, and they are well outside of the fields for the proposed radiation. Neither jejunal bypass or the esophagogastrostomy bypass using gastric fundus have any of the above advantages and are generally not used in this circumstance. If the colon is unsatisfactory for a substernal colon interposition, an attempt is made to intubate the esophagus with a traction type tube, to be followed postoperatively by radical radiation. If a tube cannot easily be placed across the lesion, then radical radiation alone is employed with hopes of achieving adequate relief of the dysphagia, reserving the option of dilatation of the lesion and peroral placement of a pulsion type tube after radiation if the dysphagia persists. In these large unresectable tumors, relief of dysphagia is less frequently achieved by radiation than with smaller lesions and recurrence of dysphagia from tumor recurrence or stricture is more common (112, 113), thus the reason for an aggressive operative approach to palliate the dysphagia at the time of the original exploration.

If there is only minimal dysphagia from an unresectable primary carcinoma without metastases, no immediate palliative procedure is indicated and radical radiation is given to the primary lesion as above with the option for later procedures to relieve dysphagia if it occurs.

Radiation is not employed if the unresectable primary lesion is visible by bronchoscopy invading to or through the mucosa of the tracheobronchial tree, because of the very frequent occurrence of an esophagorespiratory fistula as tumor necrosis occurs secondary to the radiation. Such lesions may eventually lead to esophagorespiratory fistulae, but such development is certainly accelerated by radiation.

Resectable Primary Carcinoma with no Detectable Metastases: This group of patients has the most favorable prognosis of all, and radical resection of the primary and all regional node bearing tissue en bloc is recommended. We generally perform the radical resection as described by Logan (177) which includes a formal mediastinal resection of the esophagus and all surrounding nodes to the level of the aortic arch, the gastric cardia, and lesser curvature of the stomach including all nodal tissue to the celiac axis, and resection of the spleen and distal pancreas with their intimate nodal tissue. Continuity is reestablished by esophagogastrostomy.

If the lesion is a squamous carcinoma of the distal esophagus without extension across the cardia and there is no nodal involvement within the abdomen by biopsy, we omit the splenectomy and distal pancreatectomy from the radical resection. If there is extensive involvement of the stomach by the primary carcinoma (usually an adenocarcinoma), then a total gastrectomy is performed along with the radical resection and continuity is reestablished by a Roux-en-Y esophagojejunostomy.

Postoperative radiation after radical resection may be employed if there is nodal involvement or direct tissue invasion close to the margins of resection.

Radical Resection of Carcinoma of the Distal Esophagus and Esophagogastric Junction: Technique

The Incision: Although many surgeons (178,179) recommend that all carcinomas of the esophagus be approached by separate laparotomy and right thoracotomy incisions as originally recommended by Ivor Lewis in 1946 (180), we, like Lewis and others (80,177,180-182,186), use this approach for tumors of the middle and upper thirds of the esophagus. We strongly prefer a left thoracoabdominal approach for tumors of the distal esophagus and esophagogastric junction, because of the superior exposure of the primary carcinoma and of the left upper quadrant of the abdomen allowing a much easier resection of the tissue planes necessary for a truly wide excision margin in the region of the esophagogastric junction. The only clear superiority of the right-sided approach exists when the primary carcinoma lies near or at the level of the aortic arch and tracheal bifurcation where resection from the left side is made difficult because of the aortic arch. The argument that only the right thoracic approach allows total thoracic esophagectomy if necessary is not pertinent to lower esophageal tumors because, unless the primary tumor extends to the aortic arch, the esophagus can be easily mobilized around the aortic arch from the left side and the thoracic esophagus removed as far as necessary. We have not seen the significant pulmonary compromise of the left thoracoabdominal approach as opposed to the separate laparotomy and right thoracic approach, as reported by Carey et al. (178), possibly because our incision in the diaphragm does not compromise its phrenic innervation.

With a left thoracoabdominal incision planned for definitive resection, the patient is placed in a right lateral position with the pelvis tilted back toward the supine by about 45°, but the shoulders in a full lateral position. This allows easier abdominal exploration as a preliminary to resection as previously outlined and allows better abdominal exposure later for the radical resection, yet preserving the excellent exposure of the thoracic esophagus with a posterior lateral thoracotomy. After the laparotomy has shown that resection is probably feasible, the incision is extended onto the chest wall so that one continuous incision is made beginning in the midline of the midepigastrium, across the costal arch at the seventh rib, along the course of the seventh rib below the scapula, and then upward between the scapula and spine (Fig. 26). This allows further upward extension of the incision should more superior exposure in the chest be found necessary. The left pleural cavity is now entered through the bed of the seventh rib, and exploration is done to determine if the tumor is resectable in the thorax. Unresectability is determined by subpleural fixation of the primary tumor to the

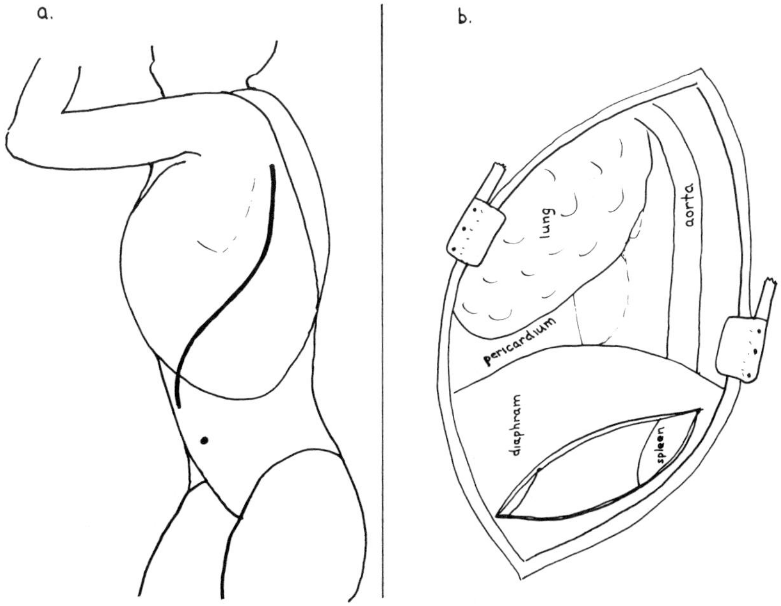

Figure 26: Left thoracoabdominal incision.

aorta, or metastatic lymph nodes outside of the resection in the superior mediastinum or lateral to the aorta. If the tumor is not resectable or if only a simple palliative resection is planned because of intraabdominal metastases, it is not necessary to divide the cartilage of the costal arch for adequate exposure. If radical resection is deemed appropriate the cartilage of the costal arch is divided and a 1 cm section removed (Fig. 27) for better reapproximation later. (If this section is not removed the cartilage tends to overlap on closure of the thoracotomy and poor healing results, whereas with this section removed, we have not seen significant problems with healing of the costal arch, a criticism some surgeons express for this incision). The diaphragm is then incised in a peripheral fashion (Fig. 28) allowing only enough rim of diaphragm on the chest wall to suture back together later during the closure of the wound. At this time, if further superior exposure is needed in the thorax, 1 cm sections of the sixth, fifth, etc. , ribs are removed posteriorly, and the intercostal bundles ligated and divided. There appears to be no added morbidity to this maneuver other than numbness in the nerve distribution which is seldom a bother to the patient. In this manner exposure from deep in the abdomen to the superior left hemithorax has been easily obtained with one continuous incision.

Radical Resection: If there is an area of concern regarding possible resectability, such as nodes at the celiac axis or primary tumor attachment to the aorta, the initial dissection should be directed to clarifying resectability in that area; otherwise, the resection should begin in the thorax and progress according to the following steps (Fig. 29):

The left inferior pulmonary ligament is resected immediately adjacent to the lung tissue up to the inferior pulmonary vein where a subadventitial plane is established reflecting the constant lymph node at the lower border of the vein toward the esophagus with the specimen. The left lung is then retracted anteriorly and superiorly, taking care not to compress the heart, and providing the exposure needed to the posterior mediastinum. The adventitial layer is dissected from the left superior pulmonary vein, the left bronchus, and the pulmonary artery, and reflected toward the esophagus.

The pleural sheath of the aorta is then incised from the diaphragm to the arch of the aorta with care to visualize and protect the left recurrent laryngeal nerve. This layer is then reflected off the anterior aorta until the right chest is entered. Several small esophageal branches will be encountered along with a frequent larger branch at the arch going to the pulmonary hilum, and they should be ligated as exposed. Otherwise this dissection is quite easy, unless the primary tumor is fixed; in

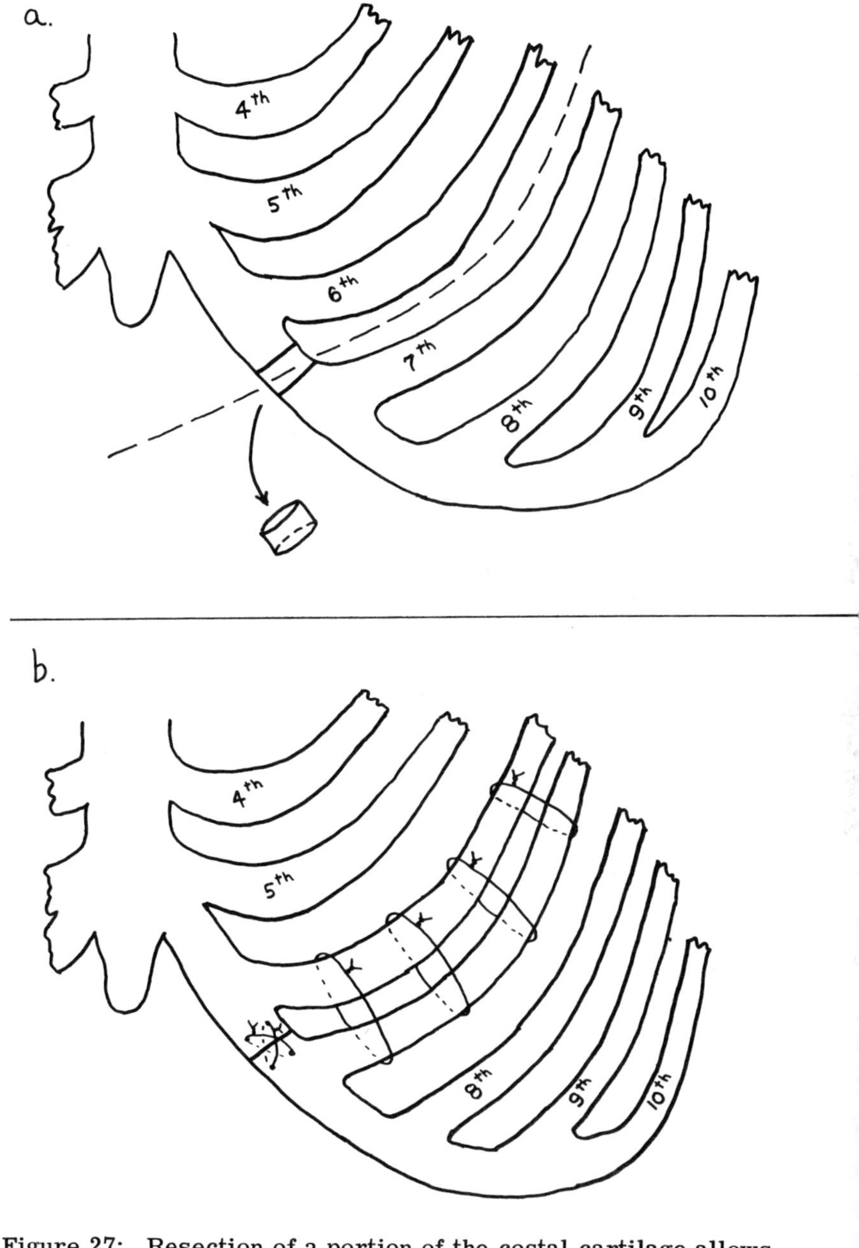

Figure 27: Resection of a portion of the costal cartilage allows better closure of the thoracoabdominal incision.

a.

b.

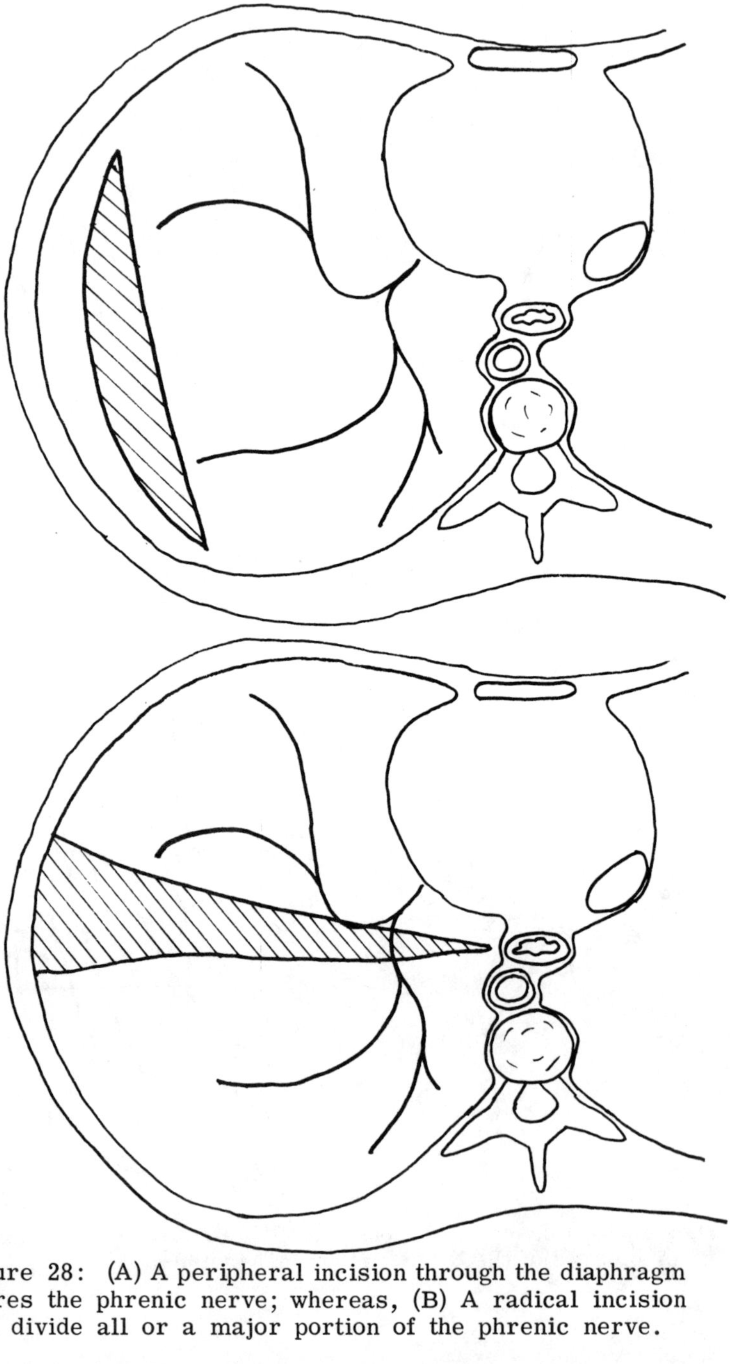

Figure 28: (A) A peripheral incision through the diaphragm spares the phrenic nerve; whereas, (B) A radical incision will divide all or a major portion of the phrenic nerve.

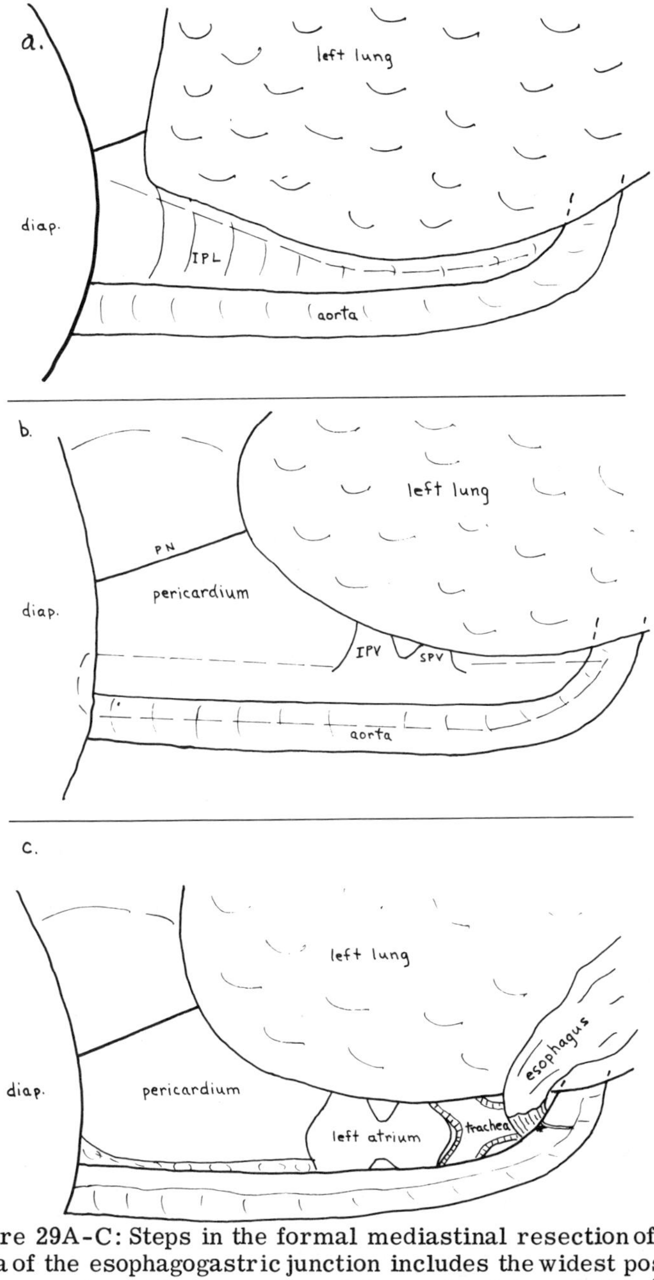

Figure 29A-C: Steps in the formal mediastinal resection of a carcinoma of the esophagogastric junction includes the widest possible margins with en bloc resection of the regional lymphatics (see text).

which case a subadventitial plane is developed which, if not easily stripped from the aorta, denotes unresectability.

Anteriorly the pleura on the pericardium is incised posterior to the phrenic nerve and reflected from the pericardium around to the right until the right chest is entered anterior to the esophagus. This dissection is carried superiorly to connect with the previous pulmonary hilar dissection. A section of pericardium is removed if involved by direct extension of the tumor.

Retracting the esophagus posteriorly, the right inferior pulmonary ligament is dissected off of the right lung up to the inferior pulmonary vein, reflecting the constant lymph node toward the specimen. This connects the subadventitial dissection of the pulmonary veins with the pleural reflection off the posterior pericardium at the left atrium. The adventitial dissection of the right superior pulmonary vein, right bronchus, and right pulmonary artery is completed, and the subcarinal group of lymph nodes are removed with the specimen. The esophagus is exposed for the first time at the aortic arch. Both vagus nerves are ligated and divided (the left vagus below the recurrent laryngeal nerve). Thus the en bloc dissection of the esophagus is complete in the mediastinum and contains a sheath around the esophagus with the widest possible resection margins containing the regional lymph nodes within the specimen (Fig. 29).

The esophageal hiatus of the diaphragm is opened further by dividing the left crux of the diaphragm. A thin rim of diaphragm is removed around the hiatus as necessary for adequate tumor margin. The thoracic duct is suture-ligated at the level of the diaphragm in the space between the aorta and the axygos vein. This latter maneuver prevents the possible occurrence of a chylothorax should the thoracic duct be injured in the dissection.

The dissection below the diaphragm (Fig. 30) is begun with mobilization of the stomach by division of the gastrocolic ligament. This is started in the midportion of the stomach and carried toward the spleen, dividing the lienocolic ligaments, then back toward the duodenum for a short distance. The lesser omentum is divided with care to avoid the right gastric artery. Total division of the gastrocolic ligament to the duodenum is not necessary for full mobilization and may risk some compromise of the blood supply to the stomach. Particular care is necessary to avoid the right gastroepiploic vein in this area. All along the greater curvature care must be taken to identify the right gastroepiploic artery and vein, since they constitute the main blood supply to the stomach to be brought up into the thorax.

The lienorenal ligament is incised and the spleen and pancreas are mobilized towards the right, in the adventitial plane posterior to the pancreas to the point where the inferior mesentery vein joins the splenic vein.

The dissection plane of the sheath of the aorta is then carried down from the mediastinum across the diaphragm to the celiac axis. The left and right inferior phrenic arteries are encountered and ligated in this dissection. The celiac nerve plexus is cut, leaving the hepatic artery branches, and the left gastric and splenic arteries are dissected free and ligated at their origins. Prior to ligation of the left gastric artery, assurance must be made that a large anomalous left hepatic artery does not arise from this vessel, and if so the ligation must be distal to that branch. The coronary vein is ligated, and the splenic vein is ligated at its junction with the inferior mesenteric vein.

The pancreas is sharply divided where the splenic and inferior mesenteric veins join. The pancreatic duct is easily visualized and is suture-ligated with a fine permanent suture. The adventitial capsule of the pancreas is reapproximated across the cut end with interrupted fine permanent sutures.

The abdominal portion of the radical resection is complete and contains all the regional lymph nodes draining the esophagogastric junction (Fig. 30).

a.

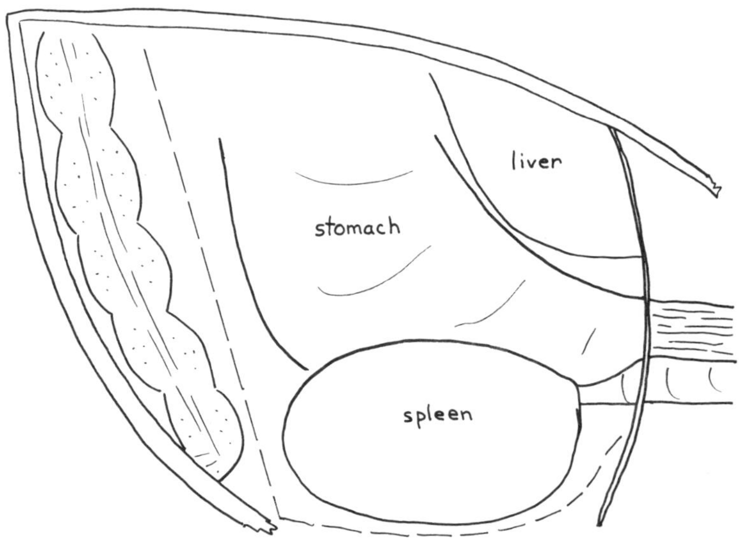

Figure 30A: First step in the formal abdominal resection of a carcinoma of the esophagogastric junction including spleen, distal pancreas, and lesser omentum with an en bloc resection of the regional lymphatics.

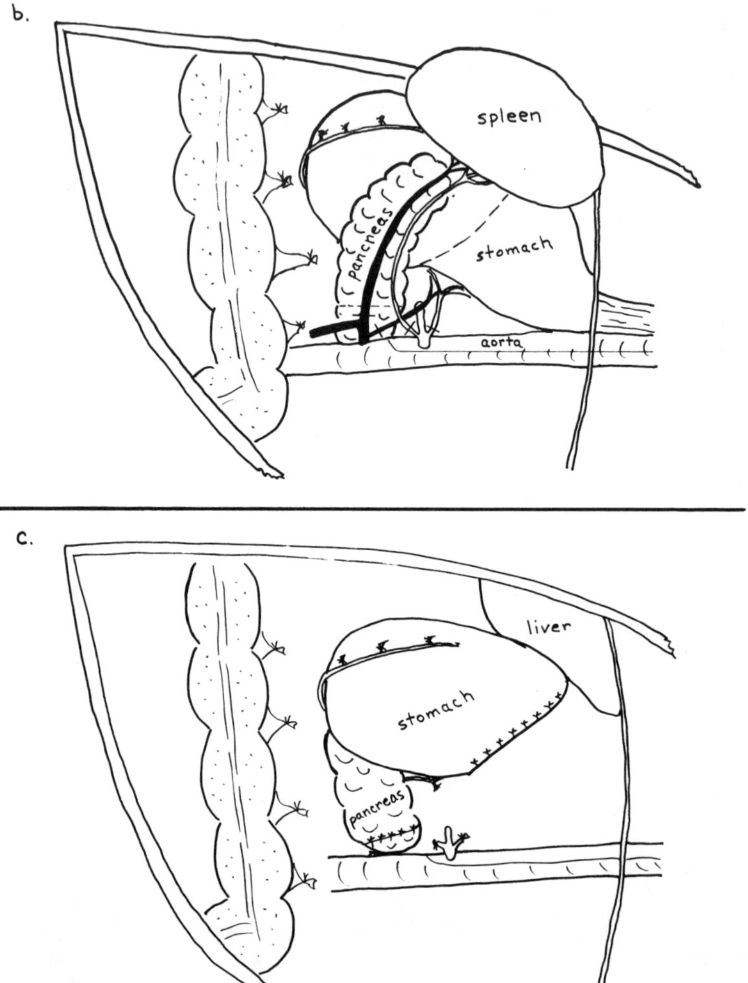

Figure 30B, C: Steps in the formal abdominal resection of a carcinoma of the esophagogastric junction including spleen, distal pancreas, and lesser omentum with an en bloc resection of the regional lymphatics.

The stomach is divided (Fig. 31), taking much of the lesser curvature to include the lymph nodes to the celiac axis and taking part of the fundus of the stomach to include the short gastric vessels and their lymph channels to the hilum of the spleen. Either the GIA or TA-90 stapler* is helpful to close the stomach. We always reinforce the staple line with an inverting row of Lambert sutures. This resection line is at least 4 cm away from gross tumor and frozen section pathology is always obtained of the resection margin to assure that it is free of carcinoma.

In squamous carcinoma, involvement of the stomach is

---

*United States Surgical Corporation.

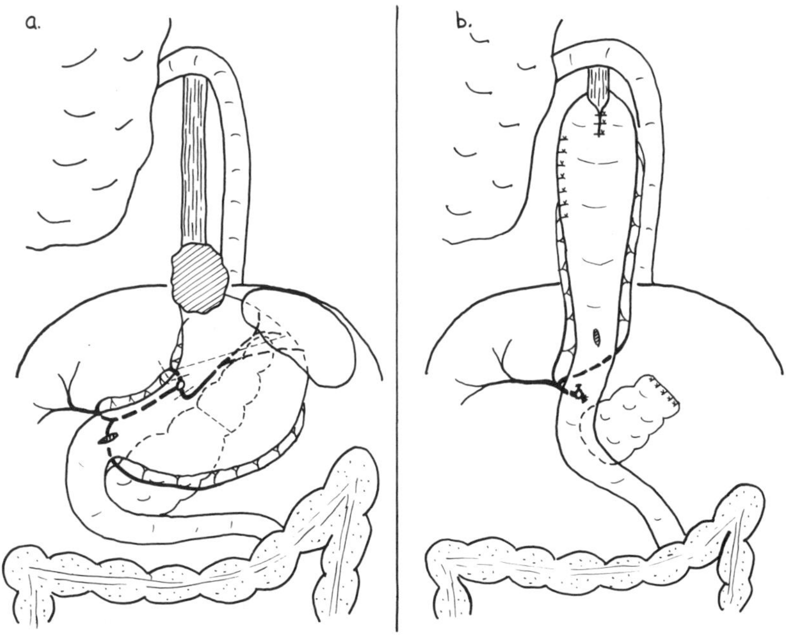

Figure 31: Resection and reconstruction of the esophagogastric junction for carcinoma. (A) Division of the stomach so that the lymphatics to the celiac axis and the hilum of the spleen and pancreas are removed en bloc with the tumor. (B) Esophagogastrostomy reconstruction with almost the entire stomach displaced into the thorax.

rarely extensive enough to require major gastric resection; however, in adenocarcinoma of the cardia, extensive infiltration of the stomach is not unusual, and there is a debate as to whether total or partial gastrectomy should be routinely performed. Several surgeons prefer total gastrectomy, but without data convincing of the necessity (184, 187). Koch (187) reviewed 46 esophagogastrectomies for adenocarcinoma of the cardia. Partial gastrectomy with esophagogastrostomy was done in 17 patients with no five-year survivals, whereas 29 total gastrectomies were done with ten five-year survivals. They, therefore, advocate routine radical total gastrectomy for adenocarcinoma of the cardia; however, careful review of their report reveals that patients who underwent partial gastrectomy had a simple resection without radical removal of the omentum, spleen, and tail of pancreas en bloc, as was performed on patients with total gastrectomy. Hawley et al. (188) reviewed 139 patients with radical resection of adenocarcinoma of the cardia including regional lymph node en bloc. Of 97 patients with partial gastrectomy, 18.6% survived five years; while 42 patients underwent total gastrectomy with a 21.4% five-year survival. The major difference in this group was between patients with no lymph node involvement versus patients with regional lymph node involvement (40.5% versus 11.8% five-year survival). Similar results have been reported by others (189, 190) who also report a slightly higher complication rate with total gastrectomy, but the difference is not significant. The most logical conclusion is that both procedures are probably equally effective if combined with an adequately radical resection of the regional lymphatics.

Our own practice is to complete a radical resection with partial gastrectomy as described, with care that the resection margin is free of carcinoma. If the residual stomach is adequate an esophagogastrostomy is fashioned. If the stomach is largely replaced by carcinoma or if the residual stomach is too small to adequately reconstruct the esophagogastric gap, a total gastrectomy is performed with radical resection of the omentum, spleen, and distal pancreas, and a Roux-en-Y esophagojejunoctomy is fashioned. Should the Roux loop prove unsatisfactory, a left colon interposition is used. The latter determination is made prior to sacrificing the stomach remnant which will be preserved for attachment of the distal colon, which seems preferable to doing a colojejunal or coloduodenal anastomosis.

The esophagus is divided at least 5 cm above the gross tumor, and again frozen section pathology is always done to assure that there is no submucosal extension of the carcinoma beyond the resection. There have been occasional cases of submucosal spread of carcinoma for long distances above a carcinoma and occasional cases of skip areas without submucosal involvement of the intervening esophagus; however, this rarely occurs when the margin is free of carcinoma at a level 5 cm above gross tumor. No hesitancy is taken to dissect the esophagus from behind the aorta in order to assure a proximal tumor-free margin. The esophageal anastomosis is then done to the left and above the aorta in such cases.

A Kocher maneuver is done of the lateral duodenum to provide further mobilization of the stomach into the chest, and a pyloromyotomy is done to prevent possible gastric stasis.

The need for division of the pyloric muscle is a very debated issue. Garlock (182), Angorn (183), and Collis (186) have led the argument that such a division is unnecessary when the stomach is to be elevated into the chest. Collis (186) further argues that such a procedure may actually be harmful in creating duodenal-gastric reflux which he feels is a major contributor to postoperative reflux esophagitis and stricture. Many others advocate routine pyloroplasty for fear of creating gastric statsis quoting an incidence of approximately 10% gastric statsis requiring reoperation if nothing is done to the pylorus. Certainly when the stomach is brought up into the chest so that there is a straight drop from the esophagus through the stomach tube to the duodenum, there appears to be little likelihood of obstruction at the pylorus, and the creation of standard Heineke-Mikulicz type pyloroplasty must decrease the potential mobility of the gastric tube upward into the chest without tension on the pyloroplasty suture line. The use of a pyloromyotomy, taking great care not to enter the duodenal mucosa, has been the compromise that we have used to avoid any possibility of disruption of a pyloroplasty incision from tension on the suture line and to assure good emptying of the gastric tube. Simple dilatation of the pyloric muscle as practiced by McCormack and Walbaum (191) may in fact be perfectly adequate.

Restoring Intestinal Continuity: Whereas resecting the tumor with an adequately radical resection to remove all carcinoma is the key to long-term control of carcinoma of the esophagogastric junction, the focal point in avoiding major complications of the surgery is focused on the reconstruction of the alimentary tract to bridge the esophagogastric defect.

Esophagogastrostomy. We, like most esophageal surgeons, prefer an esophagogastrostomy in the chest to restore intestinal continuity after esophageal resections of the esophagogastric junction for carcinoma. Unless a large amount of the stomach has been necessarily removed with the radical resection, the stomach mobilized as previously described will invariably reach high in the thorax, with the pylorus freed by the Kocher maneuver lying at the level of the esophageal hiatus. This liberal mobilization places the entire stomach in the thorax so that there is no positive abdominal pressure directly on the stomach. It allows a vertical drop of food through the stomach and pylorus with no area of dependent stomach to be adversely affected with stasis by the vagotomy. This procedure also allows ample stomach to reach the level of the transected esophagus in order to wrap the esophagogastric anastomosis with a fundoplication type of valve mechanism. This latter point is particularly important in preventing anastomotic leaks and postoperative gastroesophageal reflux. The absence of positive abdominal pressure directly on the stomach also aids in preventing gastroesophageal reflux.

Meticulous attention to detail is extremely important in creating the esophagogastric anastomosis. Probably because of its lack of a serosal covering, the esophagus does not hold sutures as well as other intestinal structures and the serosal to serosal seal present in intraabdominal intestinal anastomoses is not present to guard against small leaks. There is a tendency for downward traction on the anastomosis which must be avoided, and the exposure is often awkward particularly if the surgeon is unaccustomed to suturing at odd angles deep in the chest. The transected esophagus tends to separate into two distinct layers (Fig. 32), with the outer muscular layer retracting upward somewhat from the inner mucosal-submucosal layer. This outer muscular layer holds sutures poorly compared to the mucosal and submucosal layer, a fact of considerable importance in the creation of the anastomosis.

With these considerations in mind the following steps are pursued (Fig. 33): (1) To obtain adequate exposure the chest incision must be adequate. If the anastomosis is low beneath the aortic arch, the exposure will usually be adequate through the described seventh rib thoracoabdominal incision. If the exposure still appears awkward and particularly if the anastomosis is to be created above the aortic arch, further upward exposure may be obtained easily by the resection of 1 cm of the posterior portion of ribs six, five, etc. , and ligation of their intercostal bundles until the necessary exposure is obtained. There is very little added morbidity to this maneuver and the added exposure can be crucial to attaining a good anastomosis. The lung is retracted anteriorly and superiorly by one assistant whose entire attention should be to providing good exposure; (2) Full mobilization of the stomach must be obtained by the steps previously described so that there is no downward tension on the anastomosis. The stomach must reach to a point 5 to 6 cm above the transected esophagus without tension; (3) The most superior portion of the stomach fundus is sutured behind and at a level 4 to 5 cm above the anastomosis with several interrupted sutures between stomach and any firm surrounding tissue, such as the prevertebral fascia, aortic sheath, pericardium, adventitia of the left atrium,

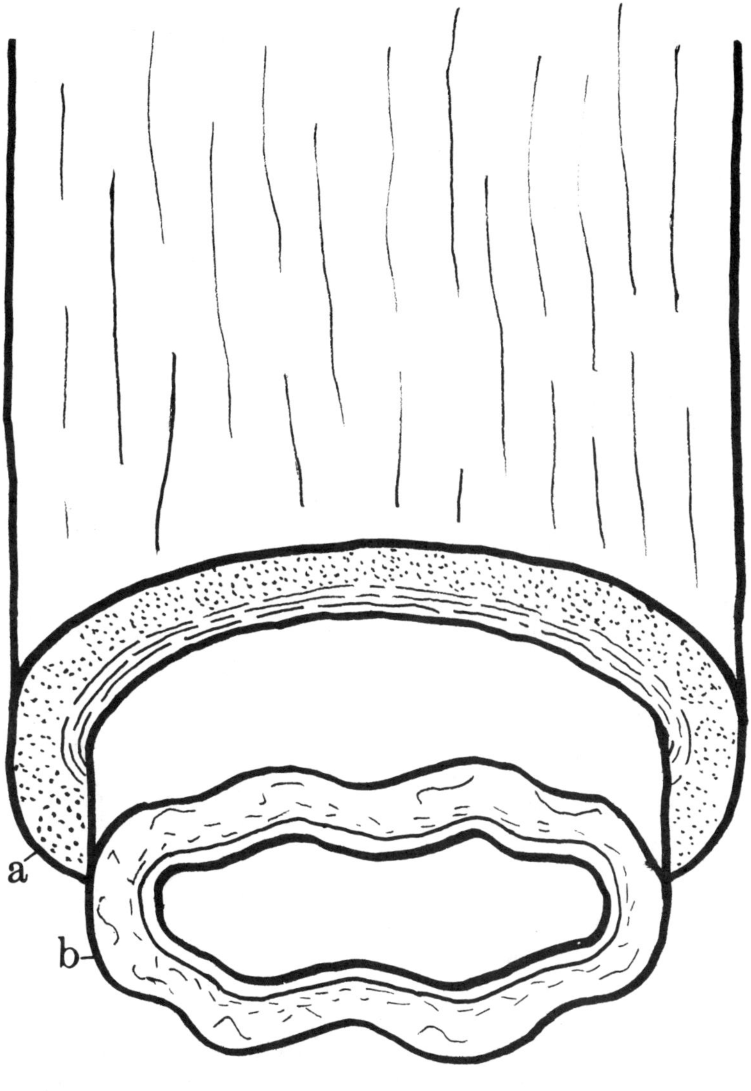

Figure 32: The transected esophagus divides into two distinct layers: (A) Outer muscular layer of both longitudinal and circular muscle which retracts upward. This layer holds sutures poorly. (B) The inner mucosal–submucosal layer which holds sutures well.

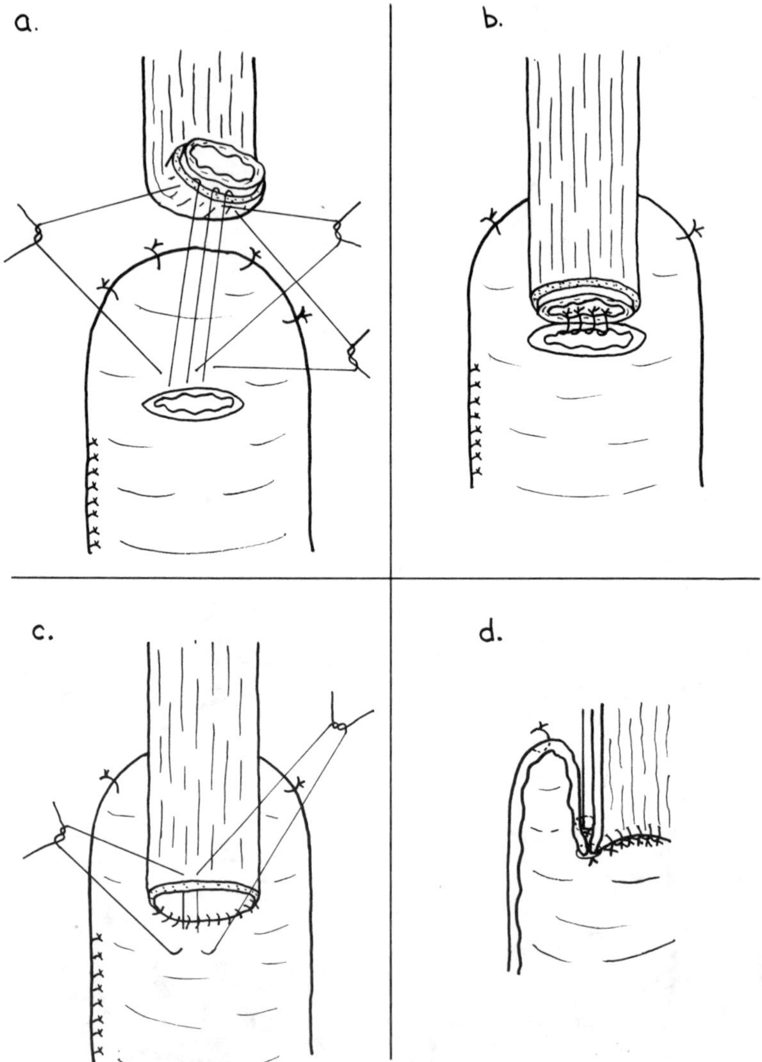

Figure 33: Steps in the esophagogastrostomy anastomosis. (A) Tacking sutures hold the weight of the stomach. Posterior outer row of sutures placed first. (B) Inner row of interrupted sutures placed carefully between the mucosal—submucosal layer of esophagus and full thickness stomach. (C) Anterior outer row of sutures between the muscular layer of esophagus and the seromuscular layer of stomach. (D) Cross-sectional detail of the suture placement.

or bronchus. The weight of the stomach should be suspended on these sutures rather than on the anastomosis; (4) A separate opening is made in the anterior wall of the stomach fundus 4 to 5 cm below the apex for the gastric side of the anastomosis. Placing the opening in the gastric resection line is to be particularly avoided because of the higher incidence of leaks, especially at the "T" where tissue viability is particularly compromised. We generally remove a 1 cm circular button of stomach musculature which immediately stretches open to 3 cm and the mucosa is then resected to effect a good opening. Small bleeders in the mucosa are carefully ligated with absorbable sutures; (5) A meticulous anastomosis is then created between the transected esophagus and the gastrotomy. Various techniques are advocated for this step. Skinner (6) strongly recommends a one layer closure of full thickness esophagus to full thickness stomach with a continuous suture of fine 5-0 wire. We, like many others (177, 179,181,182,192), prefer two layers of interrupted sutures. The outer-posterior layer of simple interrupted 4-0 nonabsorbably sutures between the muscular layer of the esophagus and the seromuscular layer of the stomach are placed 4 mm from the edge of the gastrotomy. The inner layer of synthetic absorbable (4-0 Dexon or Vicryl) sutures is placed in simple interrupted fashion between the mucosal-submucosal layer of the esophagus and full thickness stomach. All but the last two to three sutures are tied with the knots inside the lumen and the sutures are placed approximately 2 to 3 mm apart to assure a fluid-tight closure. The outer-anterior row of simple interrupted sutures are then placed with fine permanent suture material between the muscular layer of the esophagus and the seromuscular layer of the stomach. Particular care is taken to place all sutures through the tissues in a perfectly perpendicular angle with no sheering force on the needle as it passes through to avoid any tendency to lacerate at the needle holes, which can cause a small leak or fistula. A nasogastric tube is passed into the stomach pouch by direct vision just prior to the completion of the anterior-inner layer of sutures to decompress the stomach in the early postoperative period. Permanent suture material is avoided in the inner layer of the anastomosis because there is a tendency for these to cause small suture line granulations.

With the advent of the EEA stapler (United States Surgical Corporation) (193,194), interest is growing toward its use for the esophagogastrostomy anastomosis (Fig. 34). Several advantages are evident in using this instrument. The anastomosis can be created quickly; a perfect inverting anastomosis is created; and the anastomosis is done with nonreactive stainless steel staples. Use of the EEA stapler in the chest is somewhat awkward, so particular care must be taken in assuring perfect

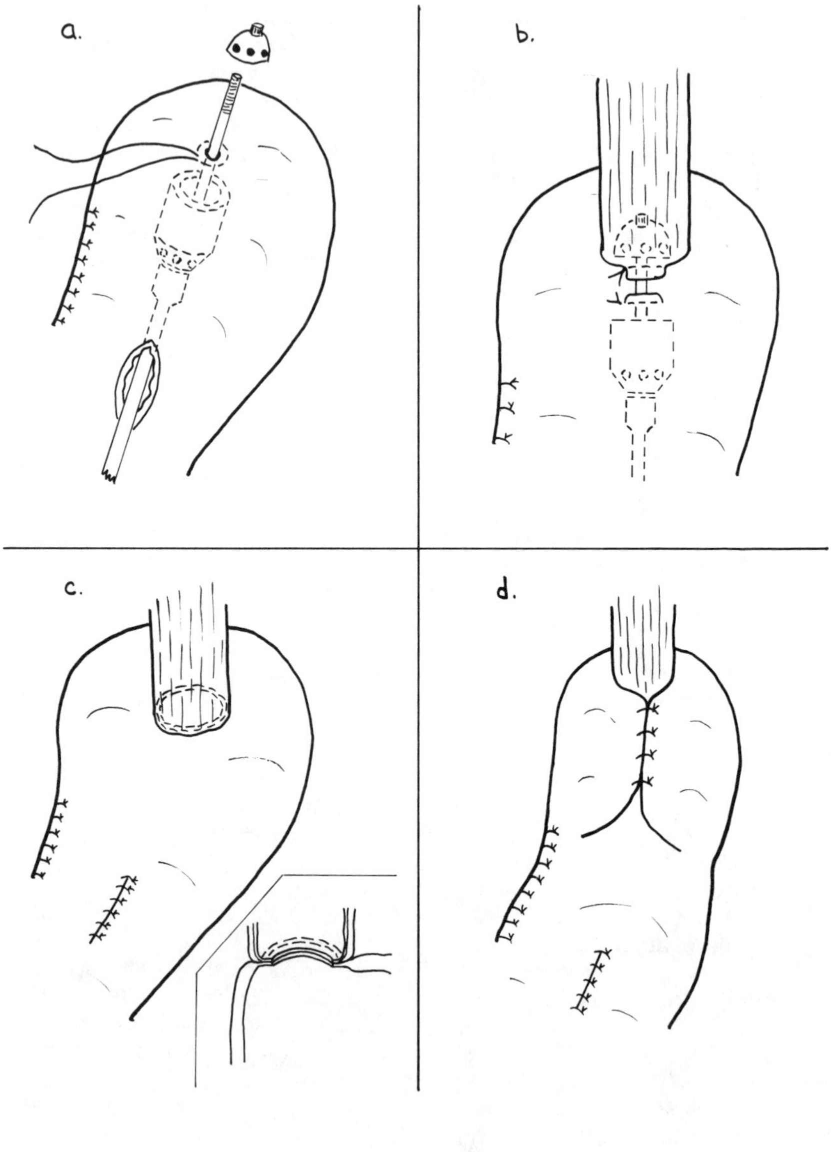

Figure 34: Use of the EEA stapler (United States Surgical Corporation) to create the esophagogastrostomy.

alignment of the tissues in the stapler or an incomplete staple line can be created which can be very difficult to repair, especially since the tendency is for the gap to occur on the posterior aspect of the anastomosis where additional sutures are very difficult to place. If the staple line is inaccurately placed and requires that the anastomosis be taken down and redone, there may be a valuable length of esophagus sacrificed and the gastrostomy may have been compromised. For these reasons, it is absolutely mandatory that the surgeon practice the use of the EEA stapler for the esophagogastrostomy anastomosis on cadavers or in the animal laboratory extensively before applying its use on patients; (6) To create a hydrostatic valve for the prevention of gastroesophageal reflux and to further reinforce the anastomosis against leak, a fundoplication around the distal esophagus is made. An inverting inkwell anastomosis with a third layer of sutures inverting the anastomosis 1 to 3 cm into the fundus of the stomach has been advocated by many. Although this inkwell effect does serve to prevent reflux to some degree, a Nissen type fundoplication as originally advocated by Bombeck et al. (195), and later by Butterfield (196, 197) has proven more effective in preventing reflux (198). To create the fundoplication (Fig. 35) the first suture is placed at a level approximately 5 cm

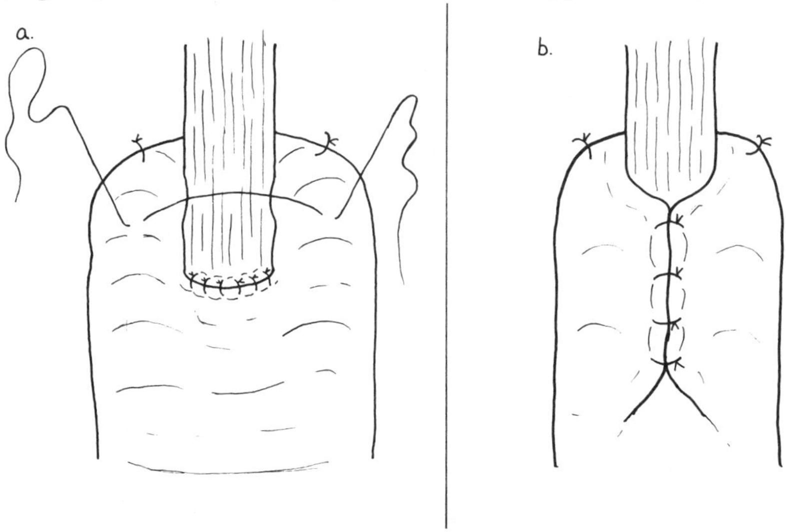

Figure 35: Creation of a fundoplication about the esophagogastrostomy to prevent gastroesophageal reflux and to further seal the anastomosis from leakage.

above the anastomosis and includes the muscular layer of the esophagus in addition to the fundus of the stomach on each side of the esophagus. The second suture is similar but 1.5 cm lower. The third and fourth sutures are in the stomach only. Care must be taken that the wrap of the fundus around the distal esophagus is not too tight. We allow two fingers alongside the esophagus. We do not pass large bougies for fear of injuring the anastomosis. This step is very important in the long-term result since reflux esophagitis and resultant strictures can be a very serious and difficult problem to manage; (7) The stomach is further suspended in the chest with sutures to the surrounding aortic adventitia and pericardium to relieve tension on the anastomosis and with sutures to the diaphragmatic hiatus which has been enlarged to accomodate the stomach and its vascular pedicle without compression. These later sutures also assure that no herniation of small or large intestine can occur alongside the stomach into the chest.

Esophagojejunostomy. When a total gastrectomy is necessary to remove the primary lesion, a Roux-en-Y esophagojejunostomy is performed to reestablish esophagointestinal continuity. Results with this technique have proven to be equal to esophagogastrostomy (188-190), so there should be no hesitancy in this decision if total gastrectomy appears desirable in the adequate removal of the primary carcinoma. Allison and da Silva (199) have well detailed the steps involved in creating a satisfactory Roux loop of jejunum for an esophagojejunostomy.

A point four to five inches from the duodenojejunal flexure is selected for the eventual point of section of the jejunum to avoid a long limb that may twist on itself (Fig. 36). The jejunum distal to this is to be used for the loop.

The most important principles in creating a long Roux loop with excellent blood supply are to carefully visualize the vascular arcade of jejunum with transilluminated light, to select a segment of jejunum which has an adequate progressive arcade of both arteries and veins, to accurately ligate these vessels at the appropriate locations, and to carefully trim the peritoneum of the mesentery to provide the greatest possible mobilization.

Transillumination of the mesentery can be achieved in a thin patient with little mesenteric fat simply by having the assistant gently hold the jejunum upward with both hands and, using the overhead operating lights aimed from the opposite side, the surgeon can easily see the vessels through the thin peritoneal covering. In a person with a fatty mesentery it may be necessary to employ a mobile sterile light in the operating field to adequately transilluminate the mesentery.

With good visualization of the mesentery, the vascular arcades are examined so that a section of jejunum of satisfactory

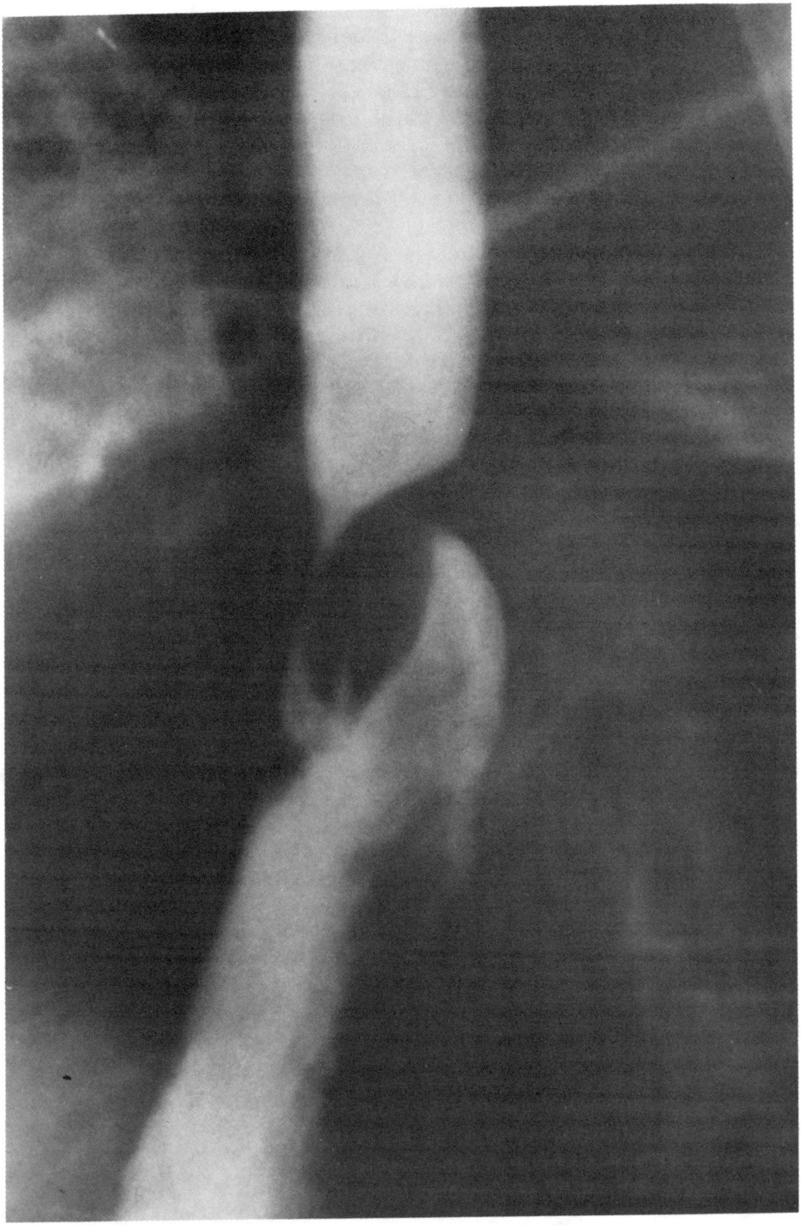

Figure 36: Barium swallow demonstrating the valve effect of a fundoplication in the thorax after esophagogastrectomy.

length is chosen that has several tiers of vascular arcades from a larger sized artery and vein progressing proximally toward the point of planned section (Fig. 37a). This section of jejunum may be slightly distal to the point four to five inches from the duodenojejunal flexure, and in that event, the short intervening segment of jejunum will be resected later.

Very accurate attention is then paid to the division of the vessels to form a progressive arcade to the jejunal loop (Fig. 37b). The peritoneum of the mesentery is divided from the point of planned section vertically down to the first peripheral arcade. The artery and vein are separately ligated with fine ligatures close to the last division leading to the jejunum. The peritoneum is then further divided down to expose the division of the next arcade where the artery and vein are again individually ligated

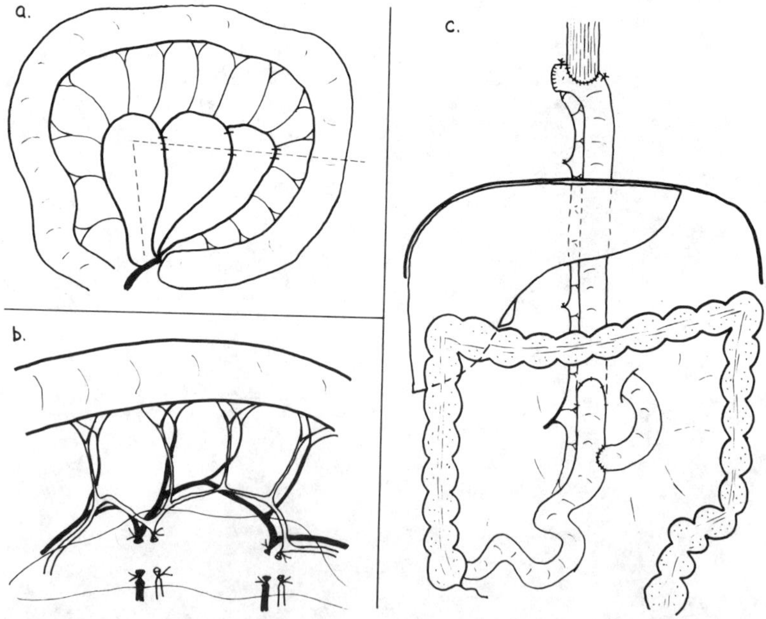

Figure 37: Steps in the creation of a Roux-en-Y jejunal loop for esophageal replacement when total gastrectomy is necessary for carcinoma at the esophagogastric junction. (A) Division of the vascular arcade to provide adequate length of jejunum. (B) Separate ligation of arteries and veins and careful division of the peritoneal mesentery at the level of the arcade to allow maximum mobilization. (C) Completed Roux loop of jejunum replacing the distal esophagus.

close to the vascular division. These steps are progressively repeated until the last and larger vessels of the lowest arcade which will supply the vascularity of the loop are exposed. Individual ligation of arteries and veins is important for as the mesentery is stretched to provide maximum length for transposition into the chest the arcades of the artery and vein tend to be somewhat different and must have separate mobility.

The height to which the jejunum may be transposed into the chest is determined not so much by the length of the intestine but by the length of the free edge of mesentery. This length can be maximized by dividing the peritoneum of the mesentery along a line closer to the intestine than the vascular arcade, so that as the loop is elongated the vascular arcade will elongate and stretch to join the peritoneal edge (Fig. 37b).

The vascular arcades tend to become larger more distal toward the middle of the jejunum, so if the length of the loop seems to be slightly inadequate, a division of a further primary vascular arcade may be justified, because the gain in overall length will probably be greater than the loss of a nonviable segment at the proximal end of the loop. This can be evaluated easily by temporarily clamping the vascular trunk with a non-crushing vascular clamp and observing the resulting extent of ischemia.

As Allison wrote (199): "The ideal Roux loop is one that reaches to the point of anastomosis exactly, without tension in its mesentery, without any surplus length, and in a straight line. The straightness of the intestine depends upon the length of its free mesenteric border being as nearly as possible equal to the length of the gut. The effective length therefore depends on the exact technique of division of peritoneum and cellular tissue, whilst the viability is governed by the care and accuracy of division of its vessels. It is important that an estimate of the required length of loop should be made at the beginning, for the risks are increased if vessels are divided unnecessarily to make too long a loop, or if a good loop is stretched only a centimeter too far and its draining vein occluded. It is equally ineffective if the limits of resection of a carcinoma, or indeed a simple oesophageal stenosis, must be governed, not by the dictates of pathology, but by the available length of a poorly constructed intestinal loop."

Once the Roux loop has been satisfactorily fashioned, the jejunum is sectioned at the planned point, the proximal end of the Roux loop is closed with an inverting two-layered closure, the jejunal loop is brought through an opening in the transverse mesocolon just to the right of the duodenojejunal flexure, and the esophagojejunal anastomosis is completed (Fig. 37c).

In creating the anastomosis between esophagus and jejunum

many of the same principles are followed as in the esophagogastrostomy. The highest point of the jejunum is suspended behind and slightly (1 cm) above the end of the esophagus with several interrupted sutures to the aortic adventitia or pericardium. A jejunal opening is made a short distance from its terminal anastomosis. The direction of this opening is determined by the exact orientation of the jejunum at the level of the anastomosis but will usually be transverse. A double-layered anastomosis identical to that described for the esophagogastrostomy is then completed with interrupted sutures using fine permanent sutures between the muscular layer of the esophagus and the seromuscular layer of the jejunum for the posterior outer layer first. This is followed by fine absorbable sutures between the mucosal-submucosal layer of the esophagus and the full thickness of jejunum for the total inner circumference. Then the completion of the anterior outer layer is made. A nasointestinal suction catheter is placed past the anastomosis into the loop prior to completion of the inner layer of sutures.

An inkwell inversion or fundoplication are not necessary since reflux does not occur up a Roux loop into the esophagus as long as the loop is at least 14 cm long.

The Y anastomosis is then fashioned by suturing the end of the proximal jejunum four to five inches beyond the ligament of Trietz to a transverse opening on the left side of the Roux loop a few inches beneath the transverse mesocolon using a double-layered inverting suture line. The mesentery of the transverse mesocolon is sutured circumferentially to the Roux loop to close the opening, and the mesentery of the proximal jejunal segment is sutured to the mesentery of the Roux loop, both to prevent internal herniation (Fig. 37C).

Colon Interposition of the Esophagus. In resecting the distal esophagus and esophagogastric junction for carcinoma, either the preferred esophagogastrostomy or esophagojejunostomy can almost invariably be used to reestablish intestinal continuity, so use of a colon interposition is only rarely necessary. We do, however, find the use of a colon interposition useful in some sitiations where an obstructing carcinoma in this location is locally unresectable but the paucity of metastatic disease makes long-term palliation a desirable goal. The detailed technique for colon interposition is, therefore, described in the section on palliative procedures. Colon interposition is often selected to restore intestinal continuity after resection of carcinomas higher in the esophagus, especially in carcinomas of the upper portion when the stomach may not reach the cervical esophagus for reconstruction.

Closure of the Wound: The left thoracoabdominal incision is closed in a routine fashion. Particular attention should be paid to the following:

1. The right chest will have been entered if a radical resection has been achieved. This is thoroughly irrigated with slightly warm saline and emptied. A separate tube is not routinely left in the right thorax since drainage freely across the mediastinum to the left side will usually be adequate.
2. A single large tube is left in a posterior-lateral position of the left chest to drain any fluid that tends to accumulate.
3. The peripheral diaphragmatic incision is closed with interrupted simple permanent sutures.
4. Positive pressure is applied to the lungs to expand any areas of atelectasis.
5. The costal margin is trimmed of a 1 cm section as previously diagramed in Fig. 27. This prevents the tendency for the ends to overlap which interferes with healing. The cartilage is then sutured with two crossed sutures of #0 Vicryl or Dexon sutures.
6. The abdominal and thoracic wounds are then closed. Our preference is for closure of the intercostal space with pericostal sutures of #1 strength. The muscular layers of the chest are closed individually with running sutures of #0 strength. The fascial layers of the abdominal portion of the incision are closed individually with interrupted sutures of 2-0. The subcutaneous tissues are reapproximated with a fine running suture, and the skin is closed with a fine subcuticular suture. Our preference for all sutures in the closure is Vicryl or Dexon, either of which offers excellent tensile strength, lasts for several weeks, yet is not a permanent suture with susceptibility to developing wound sinuses at a later time.

Postoperative Care

General Considerations

General considerations in the initial postoperative period focus attention to the status of the cardiovascular system including vascular volume and to the pulmonary system. Both of these systems sustain significant insults from the procedure of radical esophagogastrectomy, so the concerns and monitoring established in the preoperative planning are carried through the operative and the early postoperative period. The extensive dissection involved in a radical resection and reconstruction of the esophagogastric junction results in a significant extravascular accumulation of fluid similar to that seen after abdominal aortic aneurysm resection, so that particular attention is paid to accurate assessment and replacement of intravascular fluid volume. Not uncommonly this will require transfusion of several units of whole blood and/or plasma in the 24-hour period following surgery. Measurements of arterial blood pressure, central venous pressure, and urinary output usually give sufficient information to determine the adequacy of this fluid replacement; however, in many of these older patients, we have found that measurement of pulmonary artery wedge pressure which reflects the left ventricular filling pressure (a much more accurate determinant of appropriate vascular volume in older patients) and measurements of cardiac output are extremely helpful in maintaining satisfactory fluid replacement and cardiac function without overloading the vascular space (which serves as a significant additional insult to the pulmonary function which has already been somewhat compromised by the surgical incisions and the intraoperative lung retraction).

With the above considerations, we insist that the patient be transferred from the operating room to a nursing unit (recovery room or intensive care unit) where complete monitoring and respiratory care are available. Continuous monitoring of arterial blood pressure, pulse rate, and EKG, and at least hourly determinations of urine output, central venous pressure, temperature, volume loss in chest tubes and nasogastric drainage, and (when indicated) cardiac output and pulmonary artery wedge pressure are instituted. Ventilation is controlled by positive-pressure ventilation with endotracheal intubation and its adequacy determined by arterial blood gases and pH. Blood pressure is maintained at a level adequate for good coronary artery perfusion (generally 70 to 90 mmHg diastolic pressure), the central venous pressure (or preferably a pulmonary artery wedge pressure) between 10 to 15 mmHg, the cardiac index (cardiac output/m^2 of body surface) between 2 to 3 liter/min/m^2, and urine output greater than 30 ml/hr. If the arterial blood pressure or cardiac output are inadequate in spite of adequate intravascular fluid volume (CVP or PWP greater than 15 mmHg) cardiac inotropic stimulation and/or peripheral vasodilatation is achieved by the appropriate medication. Dopamine, dobutamine, or levophed are given by intravenous infusion for immediate cardiac inotropic support followed by longer-term therapy with digoxin. Dopamine and dobutamine have peripheral vasodilatation properties, but if further vasodilatation is desired, or if levophed is necessary for inotropic support, intravenous infusion of either nitroprusside or phentolamine are employed. Using these techniques of monitoring and support, the cardiovascular system can be tuned for maximum function and the smallest likelihood of complications.

Because the lungs are particularly compromised by this radical procedure and can be further insulted by any cardiovascular problem, we routinely maintain these patients on positive-pressure ventilatory support for the first 24 hours and then wean them from the respirator as tolerated by monitoring tidal volumes and the arterial pH, pCO_2, and pO_2. As soon as the respirator is discontinued and the endotracheal tube removed, vigorous respiratory hygiene is instituted by trained therapists emphasizing vigorous coughing, deep breathing exercises, postural drainage, and percussion. Nasotracheal suctioning is readily employed if deemed necessary to clear secretions.

Intravenous hyperalimentation, if begun preoperatively, is resumed throughout the operation and postoperatively until a satisfactory oral intake is assured. It is extremely important to maintain a constant rate of infusion of these solutions until good oral caloric intake is resumed. Any sudden cessation of this hyperalimentation can precipitate hypoglycemia.

The prophylactic intravenous antibiotics (generally a broad spectrum cephalosporin) begun preoperatively are continued with an intraoperative dose and also at appropriate intervals for 48 hours postoperatively.

A nasogastric tube is left in place across the anastomosis to decompress the stomach tube until intestinal activity resumes (usually three to four days). Only oral fluids in small amounts are then allowed until a barium swallow is done on day seven to ten to assure the absence of any anastomotic leak. If the anastomosis is satisfactory at that time, progression of the diet to full liquids, to soft foods, then to a normal diet is carried out over the next several days. If a small blind fistula at the anastomosis is visualized, all oral feedings are held for an additional ten days when the barium swallow is repeated.

As soon as the patient has resumed a normal diet, his incisions have shown satisfactory healing, and his general strength is adequate (generally 10 to 14 days postoperative), he is discharged from the hospital. Periodic follow-up examinations are done in the outpatient clinic with body weight determinations, physical examination, chest X-ray, hemoglobin determination, and at some later period (six weeks to six months) a repeat barium swallow. Attention is particularly focused to the possible recurrence of his carcinoma or the occurrence of the complications described in the next section.

Postoperative Complications

Postoperative complications of esophagogastrectomy for carcinoma of the distal esophagus and cardia can be categorized into early complications (within 30 days of surgery), which are generally a direct consequence of the insult of the surgical procedure, and into late complications, which are generally secondary to further spread of the primary carcinoma in spite of the surgery or secondary to physiological alterations created by the surgery.

Early Complications: Operative mortality for radical resection of the gastroesophageal junction (defined as death from any cause within 30 days of operation) varies between 2.8 to 22% in various large series (2,75,88,177,200-202,204) averaging 15.9%. Examination of the data (Table 4) reveals that most operative deaths result from three major problems: anastomotic leaks (40% of the deaths), pulmonary complications, especially pneumonia, empyema, and pulmonary emboli (20%), and cardiac complications, particularly myocardial infarction (15%).

Deaths from anastomotic leakage are particularly troubling to an esophageal surgeon, because such leakage is a direct consequence of the technical procedure. Maillard et al. (205) have examined various factors in relation to 88 anastomotic disruptions in their series of 472 resections. Malignant invasion of the resection margin carried the same incidence of disruption as no malignant invasion. Disruption occurred more frequently in resections for midesophageal lesions as opposed to distal esophageal lesions (45% versus 28%). Technical factors that significantly affected the rate of anastomotic disruption were: end-to-end esophagogastrostomy versus end-to-side anastomosis (52% versus 32%), a one-layer anastomosis versus a two or three layer anastomosis (42% versus 30%), the duration of the operation less than four hours versus greater than six hours (24% versus 55%), and whether the surgeon was considered a beginner versus an expert at the procedure (43% versus 31%). The use of preoperative hyperalimentation to achieve a positive-nitrogen balance has also been shown to decrease the incidence of anastomotic leaks in addition to wound disruption (170,171).

Pulmonary complications leading to death can be greatly decreased by careful patient selection, aggressive pre- and postoperative pulmonary care, and the prevention of intravascular overload by critical monitoring as has been outlined previously in the section on pre- and postoperative care.

Prevention of cardiac deaths is best addressed by the prevention of myocardial infarction. Experience in surgery for myocardial revascularization has clearly shown to us the value of careful monitoring of arterial blood pressure, EKG, and pulmonary artery wedge pressure in detecting the early occurrence of myocardial ischemia, and the present availability of intravenous nitroglycerine, inotropic support, and peripheral vasodilatation medications has enlarged our therapeutic responses to such ischemia when it is detected. Myocardial infarction as a cause of postoperative death after large operations in older

Table 4 Operative Mortality After Esophagogastrectomy

			Cause of Mortality			
Author	# Resections	30 Day Mortality	Anastamotic Leak	Pulmonary	Cardiac	Hemorrhage
Logan (1963)	251	21.1% (53/251)	33%			3.8%
Efskind (1965)	108	10.5% (11/108)	55%	27%	9%	9%
Zacho (1965)	85	22 % (19/85)	37%	21%	32%	
Magill & Simmons (1967)	109	11.9% (13/109)	54%			
Gunnlaugsson & Ellis (1970)	579	13.5% (78/579)	44%	19%		6%
Appelqvist (1977)	216	21.3% (46/216)	57%	15%	11%	7%
Ellis (1979)	82	2.8% (2/82)	0		100%	
Jackson (1979)	216	18 % (39/216)	13%	64%		

patients such as esophagogastrectomy for carcinoma should, therefore, decrease in frequency in the future.

Most recent authors (88,178,207) will agree with our impression that esophagogastrectomy should be performed in the present era with approximately a 5% operative mortality.

Table 5 reviews the overall major complication rate after esophagogastrectomy. Again anastomotic leaks and cardiopulmonary complications lead the list. In addition to mortality, there is a 15 to 20% reported rate of major complications.

Late Complications: The overall five-year survival after resection of carcinoma of the distal esophagus and cardia has been generally reported between 15 to 20% (2,177,200-203,208-210). More specific analysis of survival according to the microscopic cell type and the presence or absence of metastases outside of the primary lesion as demonstrated by positive versus negative lymph node involvement has been carried out by several of these authors (2,201,203,209,210) (Table 6).

Squamous cell carcinoma carried a significantly better prognosis than adenocarcinoma with overall five-year survival of 25 to 50% versus 10 to 20%. The presence of positive lymph node invasion cuts the five-year survival approximately 50% in both squamous cell carcinoma and adenocarcinoma: (45 to 80% $\longrightarrow$ 24 to 40% in squamous cell carcinoma and 20 to 60% $\longrightarrow$ 7 to 10% in adenocarcinoma). The best prognosis is clearly with squamous cell carcinoma localized to the esophagus (45 to 80% five-year survival). Squamous cell carcinoma with positive nodes has a five-year survival approximately equal to adenocarcinoma without positive lymph nodes (20 to 40%). Adenocarcinoma which has spread outside of the esophagus has the worst prognosis (7 to 9% five-year survival). Squamous cell carcinoma of distal esophagus and cardia has a better overall prognosis after resection (25 to 50% five-year survival) than squamous cell carcinoma of any other portion of the esophagus after resection or radiation (15 to 25% five-year survival); whereas adenocarcinoma of the cardia carries a slightly worse prognosis (10 to 20% five-year survival). An aggressive approach to adenocarcinoma in this location remains justified because both carcinoma in general and specifically adenocarcinoma located at the esophagogastric junction have proven to be poorly responsive to radiation therapy, the only other potentially curative therapy available at the present time.

Although some late, nonoperative related deaths occur from causes other than metastatic carcinoma, such as pneumonia, heart failure, or myocardial infarction, most of these late deaths are due to further spread of the primary carcinoma. Some recurrences cause local problems with return of dysphagia, which will be discussed in the next section, but most recurrent

Table 5 Early Mortality and Morbidity After Esophagogastrectomy

Author	# Resections	Mortality	Anastomotic leaks	Pulmonary	Cardiac	Hemorrhage	Septic	Wound	Other	Total Morbidity & Mortality
Ellis (1979)	82	2.8% (2/82)	5 % fatal 0/4-0%		2.4% fatal 2/2		1		6	16%
Stone & Wilson (1977)	52	12% (6/52)	7.7% fatal 3/4-75%	11.5% fatal 2/6	1.9% fatal 0/1				2	27%
Jackson (1979)	216	18% (39/216)	3.7% fatal 5/8-63%	21.3% fatal 26/45		1.9%		6.9%		37%

Table 6 Five-Year Survival After Resection of Carcinoma of the Distal Esophagus and Cardia

Author	# Resections	Overall 5-yr Survival	Squamous Cell Carcinoma			Adenocarcinoma		
			Overall	(+) nodes	(-) nodes	Overall	(+) nodes	(-) nodes
Sweet (1954)	109	15%						
Logan (1963)	251	16%						
Dietrich (1964)	135	15%	(7/13) 53.8%	(3/8) 37.5%	(4/5) 80%	(13/122) 10.9%	(9/102) 8.8%	(4/20) 20%
Efskind (1965)	108	12%						
Zacho (1965)	93	16%						
Magill & Simmons (1967)	109	7.4%	8.8%			6.7%		
Gunnlaugsson & Ellis (1970)	346	17.3%	(21/91) 31.9%	(10/49) 20.5%	(19/42) 45.2%	(31/245) 12.7%	(13/174) 7.5%	(18/71) 25.3%
Collis (1971)	125	16%	24.4%			11.3%		
Appelqvist (1972)	77	26%	42.8%			20.8%		

carcinoma is manifested by metastases to distant organs. The liver, lungs, adrenals, kidneys, and the general peritoneal cavity are the most common sites of metastatic spread from carcinoma of the distal esophagus and cardia. The cell type of the carcinoma does not seem to influence the pattern of spread; however, adenocarcinoma appears to metastasize somewhat earlier and more aggressively.

Other than recurrence of carcinoma leading to death, the most distressing late complication of esophagogastrectomy is a return of dysphagia due to stricture at the anastomosis. There are three likely causes of such strictures: (1) small anastomotic leaks or disruptions which are either contained locally or are drained surgically so that mediastinitis and death have not resulted but chronic inflammation of the area has eventually led to a stricture; (2) local recurrence of carcinoma in the suture line which can cause narrowing of the anastomosis or can occasionally cause dysphagia without narrowing the lumen of the anastomosis, presumably by the immobility and distortion of the bowel wall; and (3) persistent gastroesophageal reflux leading to stricture formation.

Since few authors discuss the late complications of esophagogastrectomy, the incidence of late stricture formation is difficult to accurately ascertain but probably occurs in approximately 10 to 20% of the survivors of this procedure. Since most of these strictures are the result of or are seriously aggravated by gastroesophageal reflux, the incidence of this problem must vary according to the emphasis each surgeon applies to the operative and postoperative prevention and management of gastroesophageal reflux. Collis (186) is generally unimpressed with reflux being a problem after esophagogastrectomy for carcinoma. He stresses four points: (1) reconstruction of the mediastinum so that the stomach cannot distend in the thorax; (2) no pyloroplasty to prevent retrograde duodenal reflux into the stomach; (3) all patients are required to sleep with the head of the bed propped up; and (4) the patient is required to eat six small meals a day for at least six months. Borst (211) noted a 95% incidence of esophagitis by esophagoscopy and a 10% incidence of stricture after esophagogastrectomy when the esophagogastric anastomosis was performed low in the thorax; whereas, there was 29% incidence of esophagitis and 4% incidence of stricture when the anastomosis was done high in the thorax. He concluded that positive abdominal pressure on a large intraabdominal portion of stomach contributed to the reflux and its sequelae. Fisher (179) reported no gastroesophageal reflux in 31 patients when the stomach was anastomosed high in the thorax with a fundal flap valve created by placing the fundus above and behind the anastomosis. Most recent attention has been toward recreating a true valve with a complete fundal wrap of the anastomosis and distal esophagus. Boyd (198) has shown a significant difference in incidence of symptomatic reflux, esophagitis, and stricture in 30 patients reconstructed with a fundoplication valve versus 26 patients without fundoplication. Symptomatic reflux, esophagitis, and stricture are very uncommon problems with esophagojejunostomy (212, 213), because the peristaltic section of jejunum serves as a good valve and there is no peptic fluid to regurgitate if a total gastrectomy has been performed. Although there is no significant difficulty with reflux into a colon interposition, there is a significant incidence of stricture of the proximal suture line between esophagus and colon probably due to the higher tendency of this suture line to form leaks and fistulae (211, 214).

Our general practice has been to do a full fundoplication as described previously whenever the esophagogastric anastomosis is performed below the aortic arch, particularly if a significant amount of stomach remains intraabdominal and subject to positive pressure. In high thoracic anastomoses above the aortic arch, we do a fundoplication if enough stomach is available (which is the usual case) or create a posterior flap of stomach as suggested by Fisher (179). In all cases we fully mobilize the stomach so that if possible the level of the pylorus lies at the diaphragm so that the stomach is not subject to positive pressure and there is a straight drop from the anastomosis to the duodenum.

If recurrence of dysphagia occurs after esophagogastrectomy, evaluation should include barium swallow, esophagoscopy with several biopsies of the stricture to rule out recurrent malignancy, and 24-hour pH studies of the distal esophagus (214) to note the presence and pattern of reflux. Benign stricture without reflux (generally 2° to anastomotic leak or disruption) will usually respond well to dilatation. Stricture from locally recurrent carcinoma is generally treated with radiation therapy followed by dilatation if necessary. Strictures secondary to reflux esophagitis are treated with dilatations, frequent small meals, antacids, and elevation of the bed at night. Reresection is reserved only for those patients free of metastatic carcinoma who fail to respond to these measures, and when done, includes a fundoplication if possible. If fundoplication is not possible at reexploration, serious consideration should be given to a colon interposition since patients who develop an esophageal stricture secondary to reflux that require surgical resection have a great tendency to restricture unless gastroesophageal reflux is effectively prevented. If a stricture persistently recurs in spite of these measures in a patient with metastatic carcinoma, we generally use a pulsion-type tube to palliate the dysphagia.

Chronic incisional problems can be particularly frustrating for both patient and physician. These include post thoracotomy pain, incisional hernias, and nonhealing of the costal cartilage.

Varying degrees of pain, numbness, and paresthesias occur almost universally in the incision and in the radicular distribution of the involved intercostal arteries after esophagogastrectomy. Usually this discomfort is well tolerated by the patient and rarely persists beyond six months. In persistent cases of postthoracotomy pain or paresthesias, there is usually a radicular distribution of a specific intercostal nerve. When it occurs, this type of pain can be particularly difficult to treat. Temporary and sometimes long-term relief can be obtained by intercostal block with xylocaine or marcaine and should be tried. Phenol or alcohol block is usually effective for several months but carries a significant incidence of late neuritis after six months, so it is generally reserved for patients with metastatic disease. Resection of the involved nerve, or nerve stimulator therapy may be necessary in the extreme cases. Fortunately there situations are rare.

Both incisional hernias and nonunion of the costal arch are generally preventable problems with careful attention to the wound closure, and, when they occur after proper closure, are usually related to wound infection. Incisional hernias are generally limited to the abdominal portion of the incision and are treated by the standard principles of incisional hernias. Nonunion of the costal cartilage is noted by painful motion of the cartilage and a palpable click as the cartilage ends move on each other. Cartilage has very poor resistance to infection, so in the presence of infection, reexploration should be undertaken with initial resection of the cartilage back to healthy perichondrium. If the infection persists, total resection of the cartilage may be necessary. In the absence of infection, persistent nonunion should be treated by excising a small portion of each end of the cartilage and resuturing if possible. If the ends will not come together, then resection of enough cartilage so that the ends do not rub against each other will usually stop the pain.

Certain late complications can be attributed to the vagotomy and partial or total gastrectomy. Lam (215) has shown that most patients have marked reduction in basal and maximal gastric acid output, elevated serum gastrin levels, and atropic gastritis. The mechanical response to gastric distention by food is generally retained. The dumping syndrome will occur in 10 to 20% of patients with varying combinations and degrees of weakness, nausea, epigastric distress, diarrhea, tachycardia, perspiration, flushing, and a sense of warmth occurring shortly after meals. This syndrome of symptoms is generally felt to be secondary to the rapid entrance of hypertonic food into the jejunum with a shift of fluid volume into the jejunum, jejunal dilatation, and vascular hypovolemia. Relief can usually be obtained by more frequent and smaller meals low in carbohydrates and high in proteins and fats, avoiding liquids with meals but drinking significant fluids between meals, and lying down for 20 to 30 minutes after meals. Most patients gradually recover their usual eating habits over several months without further difficulty. Diarrhea unrelated to dumping occurs in varying degrees in up to 25 to 40% of patients and usually improves markedly with time, but may require temporary oral opiate medication. Early full stomach discomfort and weight loss frequently occur and usually respond to frequent smaller meals and generally improve with time. Dumping, diarrhea, and early satistion are more common after total gastrectomy with esophagojejunostomy than after partial proximal gastrectomy.

Anemia occurring late postoperatively can be due to either iron deficiency or vitamin B12 deficiency. Since iron absorption occurs primarily in the duodenum and first portion of the jejunum, rapid transport through or bypass of this portion of the intestine can, therefore, lead to poor absorption and systemic deficiency of iron. Intrinsic factor produced in the fundus and body of the stomach is necessary for vitamin B12 absorption in the distal ileum and may be deficient in proximal gastric resection and is definitely absent in total gastrectomy. Since iron deficiency anemia is characteristically hypochromic and microcytic on microscopic examination of a blood smear, as opposed to the macrocytic anemia of vitamin B12 deficiency; specific therapy of oral iron supplements in the former and parenteral injections of vitamin B12 can be undertaken based on this simple study. In unusual or confusing cases, further studies of serum iron and iron binding capacity, bone marrow examination, and Shilling test can be done to clarify the situation. Vitamin B12 is routinely given after total gastrectomy (60 mg intramuscularly every two months). Although particular attention should be paid to the possible occurrence of late anemia after partial proximal gastrectomy, its occurrence is actually uncommon. Ward and Collis (216) reviewed 23 long-term survivors after esophagogastrectomy with esophagogastrostomy and found normal vitamin B12 and folic acid in all patients and iron deficiency anemia in only one of the 23 patients. Inberg (217) studied nine patients after esophagectomy, five patients after proximal gastrectomy, and six patients after total gastrectomy, all two to eight and one-half years postoperatively. He found pathologically low levels of vitamin B12 in all patients after total gastrectomy and in two of five patients after proximal gastrectomy. Shilling test was abnormal in all patients with total or proximal gastrectomy and in two of nine patients after esophagectomy. Iron absorption and bone marrow studies were normal in most patients as was folate absorption. Slight anemia was present in only six patients. The other patients had normal hemoglobins, showing that the vitamin B12 deficiency after gastrectomy may not be readily apparent particularly early.

Chapter 5

SUMMARY AND PROGNOSIS

Our goal in this treatise on gastroesophageal carcinoma has been: (1) to clearly define the rationale for considering carcinoma of the distal esophagus and the cardia of the stomach as a distinct clinical entity separate from carcinoma of the remainder of the esophagus and of the remainder of stomach; (2) to describe the known factors in the etiology of these tumors; (3) to fully describe the natural history of these carcinomas both with and without treatment; (4) to delineate the usual clinical manifestations and the steps in the diagnosis of gastroesophageal carcinoma; and (5) to describe fully our approach to selective therapy of these carcinomas based on individual patient circumstance and accurate staging of the spread of the disease.

We have discussed the relative merits of radiation, radiation plus surgical resection, surgical resection alone, chemotherapy, and various forms of palliative therapy in the treatment of carcinoma of the esophagogastric junction. We have presented a selective therapy scheme which details our preference and rationale for therapy in algorithmic form to show the stepwise process we use to arrive at the preferred therapy in each specific clinical situation. The central role of exploratory laparotomy is stressed as the crucial step in determining the actual pathological stage of the disease and the resectability of the primary carcinoma, determinations which in the majority of patients lead to the immediate choice of appropriate therapy.

The various surgical techniques used to treat carcinoma at the gastroesophageal junction have been described in detail, including palliative prosthetic intubation, colon interposition, simple esophagogastric bypass, simple and radical esophagogastrectomy, and jejunal interposition. In addition to the exact technical details of each surgical procedure, we have particularly stressed the role each procedure plays in selective therapy and its expected results and complications.

Although carcinoma of the gastroesophageal junction

generally carries a grave prognosis, hopefully we have conveyed to the reader that an aggressive approach to diagnosis and treatment is rewarded by valued palliation of desperate symptoms in most patients and long-term control of cancer in many. Further improvement in the overall results with carcinoma of the gastroesophageal junction will not come from a single point of attack but must be based on several approaches. Prevention of the disease must be the most crucial direction toward improvement. As detailed in the section on etiology and epidemiology, a great deal is being learned about dietary factors in carcinoma of the esophagus and stomach. Of particular interest and probable future importance is the role of the nitrosamines and nitrosamides. Hopefully this relationship of dietary factors will soon be further clarified to a point of allowing a preventative dietary approach.

Earlier diagnosis is the second most important point of attack for future gains on this disease. This requires education of the public to report symptoms of dysphagia early and further education of physicians to treat any symptom of dysphagia, particularly in any person over 50 years of age, as a grave symptom warranting a rapid and thorough investigation. Gains in the treatment of gastroesophageal carcinoma must come first in more general application of aggressive therapy as we have outlined it here, emphasizing the use of preoperative hyperalimentation, critical monitoring, and careful surgical technique to improve the surgical mortality rate of radical esophagogastrectomy. Further improvements in therapy will most likely come from improving our results in stage II and stage III disease by combining aggressive multiple drug chemotherapy with surgical resection or radiation. As success increases in the use of chemotherapeutic regimens hopefully we will begin to use the term long-term control of disease in place of cure as a truly valid concept in gastroesophageal carcinoma.

REFERENCES

1. Magill, T.G. and Simmons, R.L. Resection of Cardio-esophageal Carcinoma. Arch Surg 94:865-870, 1967.

2. Gunnlaugsson, G.H., Wychulis, A.R., Roland, C. and Ellis, F.H. Analysis of the Records of 1657 Patients with Carcinoma of the Esophagus and Cardia of the Stomach. Surg Gynecol Obstet 130:997-1005, 1970.

3. Sefton, G.K., Cooper, D.J., Grech, P. and Giddings, A. E.B. Assessment and Resection of Carcinoma at the Gastroesophageal Junction. Surg Gynecol Obstet 144:563-566, 1977.

4. Stone, R., Rangel, D.M., Gordon, H.E. and Wilson, S.E. Carcinoma of the Gastroesophageal Junction: A Ten Year Experience with Esophagogastrectomy. Am J Surg 134:70-76, 1977.

5. Burgess, H.M., Baggenstoss, A.H., Moersch, H.J. and Clagett, O.T. Carcinoma of the Esophagus: A Clinico-Pathologic Study. Surg Clin North Am 31:965-976, 1951.

6. Skinner, D.B. Esophageal Malignancies: Experience with 110 Cases. Surg Clin North Am 56:137-147, 1976.

7. Van Andel, J.G., Dees, J., Dijkhuis, C.M., Fokkens, W., Van Houten, H., De Jong, P.C. and Woerkom-Eykenbom, WMH. Carcinoma of the Esophagus: Results of Treatment. Ann Surg 190:684-689, 1979.

8. Clarke, J.S., Cruze, K., Farra, S.E. and Longmire, W. P. Jr. The Natural History and Results of Surgical Therapy for Carcinoma of the Stomach: An Analysis of 250 Cases. Am J Surg 102:143, 1961.

9. Cassell, P. and Robinson, J.O. Cancer of the Stomach: A Review of 854 Cases. Br J Surg 603-607, 1976.

10. Inberg, M.V., Vuori, J. and Viikari, S.J. Carcinoma of the Stomach: A Follow-up Study of 1963 Patients. Acta Chir Scand 138:195-201, 1972.

11. Raphael, H. A., Ellis, F. H. and Dockerty, M. B. Primary Adenocarcinoma of the Esophagus: 18 Year Review and Review of the Literature. Ann Surg 164:785-796, 1966.

12. Turnbull, A. D. and Goodner, J. T. Primary Adenocarcinoma of the Esophagus. Cancer 22:915-918, 1968.

13. Ackerman, L. V. and del Regato, J. O., ed. Cancer: Diagnosis, Treatment and Prognosis. C. V. Mosby, St. Louis, 1970, pp. 430-435.

14. Nissan, S., Bar-Moar, J. A. and Levy, E. Lymphosarcoma of the Esophagus: A Case Report. Cancer 34:1321-1323, 1974.

15. Matsusaka, T., Watanabe, H. and Enjoji, M. Anaplastic Carcinoma of the Esophagus. Cancer 37:1352-1358, 1976.

16. Sumiyoshi, A., Sannoe, Y. and Tanaka, K. Rhabdomyosarcoma of the Esophagus: A Case Report. Acta Pathol Jap 22: 581-589, 1972.

17. De Meester, T. R. and Skinner, D. B. Polypoid Sarcomas of the Esophagus: A Rare but Potentially Curable Neoplasm. Ann Thorac Surg 20:405-415, 1975.

18. Matsusaka, T., Watanabe, H. and Enjoji, M. Pseudosarcoma and Carcinosarcoma of the Esophagus. Cancer 37: 1546-1555, 1976.

19. Freant, L., Levin, R., Peabody, J. and Absolon, K. Primary Adenoid Cystic Carcinoma of the Esophagus. J Thorac Cardiovasc Surg 69:785-789, 1975.

20. Weitzner, S. Mucoepidermoid Carcinoma of the Esophagus. Arch Pathol 90:271-273, 1970.

21. Silverberg, E. Cancer Statistics: 1980. CA 30 (1):23-38, 1980.

22. Langman, M. J. S. Epidemiology of Cancer of the Oesophagus and Stomach. Br J Surg 58:792-793, 1971.

23. Haenszel, W. and Correa, P. Developments in the Epidemiology of Stomach Cancer over the Past Decade. Cancer Res 35:3452-3459, 1975.

24. Oesophageal Cancer in China. Br Med J 3:61, 1975.

25. Mahboubi, E. Epidemiologic Study of Esophageal Carcinoma in Iran. Int Surg 56:68-71, 1971.

26. Hormozdiari, H., Day, N. E., Aramesh, B. and Mahboubi, E. Dietary Factors and Esophageal Cancer in the Caspian Littoral of Iran. Cancer Res 35:3493-3498, 1975.

27. Day, N. E. Some Aspects of the Epidemiology of Esophageal Cancer. Cancer Res 35:3304-3307, 1975.

28. Young, J. L., Denesa, S. S. and Cutler, S. J. Incidence of Cancer in United States Blacks. Cancer Res 35:3523-3536, 1975.

29. Audiger, J. C., Tuyns, A. J. and Lambert, R. Epidemiology of Oesophageal Cancer in France. Digestion 13:209-219, 1975.

30. Schonland, M. and Bradshaw, E. Oesophageal Cancer in Natal Bantu: A Review of 516 Cases. S Afr Med J 43:1028-1031, 1969.

31. Sterup, K. and Mosbech, J. Sex Ratio of Gastric Cancer Related to Site of the Tumour. Scand J Gastroenterol 9:87-89, 1974.

32. MacDonald, W. C. Clinical and Pathologic Features of Adenocarcinoma of the Gastric Cardia. Cancer 29:724-732, 1972.

33. Haenszel, W., Kurihara, M., Segi, M. and Lee, R. K. C. Stomach Cancer Among Japanese in Hawaii. J Natl Cancer Inst 49:969-988, 1972.

34. Hirayama, T. Epidemiology of Cancer of the Stomach with Special Reference to Its Recent Decrease in Japan. Cancer Res 35:3460-3463, 1975.

35. Schoenberg, B. S., Bailar, J. C., III and Fraumeni, J. F. Cancer Mortality Patterns of Esophageal Cancer in the United States, 1930-1967. J Natl Cancer Inst 46:63-73, 1971.

36. Lynch, H. T., Ewers, D. D., Krush, A. J., Sharp, E. A. and Swartz, M. J. Esophageal Cancer in a Midwestern Community. Am J Gastroenterol 55:437-442, 1971.

37. Bradshaw, E. and Schonland, M. Smoking, Drinking, and Oesophageal Cancer in African Males of Johannesburg, South Africa. Br J Cancer 30:157-163, 1974.

38. De Jong, U., Breslow, N., Goh Ewe Hong, J., Sridharan, M. and Shanmugaratnam, K. Aetiologic Factors in Oesophageal Cancer in Singapore Chinese. Int J Cancer 13:291-303, 1974.

39. Kmet, J. and Mahboubi, E. Esophageal Cancer in the Caspian Littoral of Iran: Initial Studies. Science 175:846-853, 1972.

40. Zacho, A., Nielsen, J. and Cederqvist, C. Relationship between Type of Tobacco Used and Localization of Tumor in Patients with Gastric Cancer. Acta Chir Scand 141:676-679, 1975.

41. Flamant, R., Lassere, O., Lazar, P., Leguerinais, J., Denoix, P. and Swartz, D. Differences in Sex Ratio According to Cancer Site and Possible Relationship with Use of Tobacco and Alcohol: Review of 65,000 Cases. J Natl Cancer Inst 32:1309-1316, 1964.

42. Weisburger, J. Mechanism of Action of Diet as a Carcinogen. Cancer 43:1987-1995, 1979.

43. Graham, S., Schotz, W. and Martino, P. Alimentary Factors in the Epidemiology of Gastric Cancer. Cancer 30:927-938, 1972.

44. Hill, M. J., Hawksworth, G. and Tattersall, G. Bacteria, Nitrosamines, and Cancer of the Stomach. Br J Cancer 28:562-567, 1972.

45. Naef, A. P., Savary, M. and Ozello, L. Columnar-Lined Lower Esophagus: An Acquired Lesion with Malignant Predisposition. J Thorac Cardiovasc Surg 70:826-835, 1975.

46. Stalsberg, H. and Taksdal, S. Stomach Cancer Following Gastric Surgery for Benign Conditions. Lancet 2:1175-1177, 1971.

47. Schrumpf, E., Stadaas, J., Myren, J., Serck-Hanssen, A.S., Aune, S. and Osnes, M. Mucosal Changes in the Gastric Stump 20-25 Years After Partial Gastrectomy. Lancet 2:467-469, 1977.

48. Nicholls, J.C. Carcinoma of the Stomach Following Partial Gastrectomy for Benign Gastroduodenal Lesions. Br J Surg 61:244-249, 1974.

49. MacGregor, I.L. Carcinoma of the Colon and Stomach: A Review with Comment on Epidemiologic Associations. JAMA 227:911-915, 1974.

50. Wychulis, A.R., Woolam, G.L., Anderson, H.A. and Ellis, F.H. Achalasia and Carcinoma of the Esophagus. JAMA 215:1638-1641, 1971.

51. Hankins, J.R. and McLaughlin, J.S. The Association of Carcinoma of the Esophagus with Achalasia. J Thorac Cardiovasc Surg 69:355-360, 1975.

52. Lortat-Jacob, J.L., Richard, C.A., Fekete, F. and Testart, J. Cardiospasm and Esophageal Carcinoma: Report of 24 Cases. Surgery 66:969-975, 1969.

53. Postlethwait, R.W. Surgery of the Esophagus. New York: Appleton-Century-Crofts, 1979.

54. Johnson, R.G. and Monroe, L.S. Carcinoma of the Esophagus Developing in Progressive Systemic Sclerosis. Gastrointest Endosc 19:189-191, 1973.

55. Fujimura, S., Dogura, K., Sugimura, T. and Takayama, S. The Effect of Limited Administration of N-Methyl-N'-Nitroso-N-Nitrosoguanidine on the Induction of Stomach Cancer in Rats. Cancer Res 30:842-848, 1970.

56. Sugimura, T., Tanaka, N., Kawachi, T., Kogure, K., Fujimura, S. and Shimosato, Y. Production of Stomach Cancer in Dogs by N-Methyl-N'-Nitroso-N-Nitrosoguanidine. Gann 62:67, 1971.

57. Baker, J.R., Mason, M.M., Yerganian, G., Weisburger, E.K. and Weisburger, J.M. Induction of Tumors of the Stomach and Esophagus in Inbred Chinese Hamsters by Oral Diethylnitrosamine. Proc Soc Exp Biol Med 146:291-293, 1974.

58. Nakamura, T., Matsuyama, M. and Kishimoto, H. Tumors of the Esophagus and Duodenum Induced in Mice by Oral Administration of N-Ethyl-N'-Nitro-N-Nitrosoguanidine. J Natl Cancer Inst 52:519-522, 1974.

59. Sekizuka, H., Doi, H., Sunagawa, M., Nagai, S., Kojima, S., Hiraide, H., Hoshi, K. and Murakami, T. Induction of Esophageal Cancer Associated with Gastric Cancer in a Dog by N-Ethyl-N'-Nitro-N-Nitrosoguanidine. Gann 66:683-688, 1975.

60. Reuber, M.D. Effect of Age and Sex on Lesions of the Esophagus in Buffalo Strain Rats Ingesting Diethylnitrosamine. Exp Cell Res 44:65-72, 1976.

61. Hoffman, D., Adams, J.D., Brunneman, K.D. and Hecht, S.S. Assessment of Tobacco-specific N-Nitrosamines in Tobacco Products. Cancer Res 39:2505-2509, 1979.

62. Spiegelhalder, B., Eisenbrand, G. and Preussman, R. Contamination of Beer with Trace Quantities of N-Nitrosodimethylamine. Food Cosmet Toxicol 17:29-31, 1979.

63. Pignatelli, B., Castenegro, M. and Walker, E.A. Effects of Gallic Acid and of Ethanol on Formation of Nitrosodiethylamine. IARC Sci Publ 14:173-178, 1976.

64. Lieber, C.A., Seitz, H.K. Garro, A.J. and Wormer, T. M. Alcohol-related Diseases and Carcinogenesis. Cancer Res 39:2863-2886, 1979.

65. Roach, W.A. An Attempt on a Cause and Prevention of Oesophageal Cancer in The Transkei Bantu. S Afr Med J 47:347-348, 1973.

66. Mirvish, S.S. Kinetics of Nitrosamide Formation from Alkylureas, N-Alkylurethans and Alkylguanidines: Possible Implications for the Etiology of Human Gastric Cancer. J Natl Cancer Inst 46:1183-1193, 1971.

67. Mirvish, S.S., Wallcove, L., Eagen, M. and Shubik, P. Ascorbate-Nitrite Reaction: Possible Means of Blocking the Formation of Carcinogenic N-Nitroso Compounds. Science 177:65-68, 1972.

68. Endo, H. and Takahashi, K. Methylguanidine, a Naturally Occurring Compound Showing Mutagenicity After Nitrosation in Gastric Juice. Nature 245:325-326, 1973.

69. Bayland, E. and Walker, S. A. Effect of Thiocyanate on Nitrosation of Amines. Nature 248:601-602, 1974.

70. Weisburger, J. H. and Raineri, R. Dietary Factors and the Etiology of Gastric Cancer. Cancer Res 35:3469-3474, 1975.

71. Kawamura, T., Sakai, K., Miyasama, F. Studies on Nitrosamines in Foods (IV): Distribution of Secondary Amines in Foods. J Food Hyg Soc Jap 12:192-197, 1971.

72. Fong, Y. Y. and Walsh, E. O. F. Carcinogenic Nitrosamines in Cantonese Salt-Dried Fish. Lancet 6 Nov: 1032, 1971.

73. MacDonald, W. C., Anderson, F. H. and Hashimoto, S. Histologic Effect of Certain Pickles on the Human Gastric Mucosa: A Preliminary Report. Can Med Assoc J 96:1521-1525, 1967.

74. Ruddell, W. S. J., Bone, E. S., Hill, M. J., Blendis, L. M. and Walters, C. L. Gastric Juice Nitrite: A Risk Factor for Cancer in the Hypochlorhydric Stomach. Lancet 2:1037-1039, 1976.

75. Appelqvist, P. Carcinoma of the Oesophagus and Gastric Cardia. Acta Chir Scand (Suppl) 430:1-92, 1972.

76. Alrenga, D. P. Fatal Hemorrhage Complicating Carcinoma of the Esophagus. Gastroenterology 65:422-426, 1976.

77. Gelzand, E. A., Braucher, R. E. and Kirsner, J. B. Aortic Perforation Complicating Carcinoma of the Esophagus. Endoscopy 14:36-39, 1967.

78. Scanlon, E. F., Morton, D. R., Walker, J. M. and Watson, W. L. The Case Against Segmental Resection for Esophageal Carcinoma. Surg Gynecol Obstet 101:290-296, 1955.

79. Sunderland, D. A., McNeer, G., Ortega, L. G. and Pearce, L. S. The Lymphatic Spread of Gastric Cancer. Cancer 6:987-996, 1953.

80. Berry, R. E. L. and Rottschager, W. The Lymphatic Spread of Cancer of the Stomach Observed in Operative Specimens Removed by Radical Surgery Including Total Pancreatectomy. Surg Gynecol Obstet 104:269-279, 1957.

81. Majima, S., Harada, M. and Etani, S. End Results of Gastrectomy for Gastric Cancer: Effect of Extensive Lymph Node Dissection. Surgery 68:753-758, 1970.

82. Hankins, J. R., Cole, F. N., Attar, S. Frost, J. L. and McLaughlin, J. S. Adenocarcinoma Involving the Esophagus. J Thorac Cardiovasc Surg 68:148-158, 1974.

83. Younghusband, J. D. and Aluwihare, A. P. R. Carcinoma of the Oesophagus: Factors Influencing Survival. Br J Surg 57:422-430, 1970.

84. Cedermark, B. J., Blumenson, L. E., Pickren, J. W. and Elias, E. G. The Significance of Metastases to the Adrenal Gland from Carcinoma of the Stomach and Esophagus. Surg Gynecol Obstet 145:41-48, 1977.

85. Goodner, J. T. and Turnbull, A. D. M. Bone Metastases in Cancer of the Esophagus. Am J Roent Rad Ther Nucl Med 111:365-367, 1971.

86. Stephens, R. L., Hansen, H. H. and Muggia, F. M. Hypercalcemia in Epidermoid Tumors of the Head and Neck and Esophagus. Cancer 31:1487-1491, 1973.

87. Chandrasekhara, R., Pilz, C. G. and Levitan, R. Hypercalcemia Associated with Esophageal Carcinoma in the Absence of Bone Metastases. Am J Dig Dis 20:173-175, 1975.

88. Ellis, F. H. and Gibb, S. Esophagogastrectomy of Carcinoma: Current Hospital Mortality and Morbidity Rates. Ann Surg 190:699-705, 1979.

89. American Joint Committee for Cancer Staging and End-Results Reporting: Manual for Staging of Cancer 1979. Chicago. Whiting Press, 1979.

90. Hankins, J. R., Cole, F. N., Ward, A., Carter, E. A., Weiner, S. and McLaughlin, J. S. Carcinoma of the Esophagus: The Philosophy for Palliation. Ann Thorac Surg 14:189-197, 1972.

91. Clinical Staging System for Carcinoma of the Esophagus. CA 25:50-57, 1975.

92. Duvoisin, G. E., Ellis, F. H. and Payne, W. S. The Value of Palliative Prostheses in Malignant Lesions of the Esophagus. Surg Clin North Am 47:827-831, 1967.

93. Zimmerman, J. M. and King, T. C. Use of the Souttar Tube in Management of Advanced Esophageal Cancer. Ann Surg 169:867-872, 1969.

94. Bertelson, S. Palliative Treatment of Obstructing Neoplasia of the Oesophagus and Cardia by Permanent Intubation. Acta Chir Scand 137:165-168, 1971.

95. Pringle, R. and Winsey, H. S. The Palliation of Oesophageal Carcinoma. J R Coll Surg Edinb 18:188-190, 1973.

96. Le Roux, B. T. The Influence of Resection on the Natural History of Carcinoma of the Hypopharynx, Esophagus, and Proximal Stomach. Surg Gynecol Obstet 115:162-174, 1967.

97. Ammann, J. F. and Collis, J. L. Palliative Intubation of the Esophagus: Analysis of 59 Cases. J Thorac Cardiovasc Surg 61:863-869, 1971.

98. Bruni, H. C. and Nelson, R. S. Carcinoma of the Esophagus and Cardia: Diagnostic Evaluation in 113 Cases. J Thorac Cardiovasc Surg 70:367-370, 1975.

99. Wiot, J. W. and Felson, B. Esophageal Cancer: Radiographic Differential Diagnosis. JAMA 226:1548-1552, 1973.

100. Morrissey, J. F. Endoscopic Diagnosis. JAMA 226:1552-1554, 1973.

101. Winawer, S. J., Sherlock, P., Belladonna, J. A., Melamed, M. and Beattie, E. J. Endoscopic Brush Cytology in Esophageal Cancer. JAMA 232:1358, 1975.

102. Akiyama, H., Kogure, T. and Itai, Y. The Esophageal Axis and Its Relationship to the Resectability of Carcinoma of the Esophagus. Ann Surg 176:30-36, 1972.

103. Murray, G. F., Wilcox, B. R. and Starek, P. J. K. The Assessment of Operability of Esophageal Carcinoma. Ann Thorac Surg 23:393-399, 1977.

104. Berglin, E., Groth, J. and William-Olsson, G. Mediastinoscopy in Cancer of the Esophagus or Cardia. Scand J Thorac Cardiovasc Surg 11:275-277, 1977.

105. Fee, H.J., Holmes, E.C., Gewirtz, H.S., Ramming, K. P. and Alexander, J.M. Role of Pulmonary Vascular Resistance Measurements in Preoperative Evaluation of Candidates for Pulmonary Resection. J Thorac Cardiovasc Surg 75:519-523, 1978.

106. Arkins, R., Smessaert, A.A. and Hicks, R.G. Mortality and Morbidity in Surgical Patients with Coronary Artery Diseases. JAMA 190:485-488, 1964.

107. Fraser, J.F.G., Ramachandran, P.R. and Davis, H.S. Anesthesia and Recent Myocardial Infarction. JAMA 199: 318-320, 1967.

108. Goldman, L. et al. Multifactorial Index of Cardiac Risk in Noncardiac Surgical Procedures. N Engl J Med 298:339-340, 1977.

109. Skinner, J.F. and Pearce, M.L. Surgical Risk in the Cardiac Patient. J Chronic Dis 17:57-59, 1964.

110. Watson, W.L. and Goodner, J.T. Radiation Treatment of Esophageal Cancer. Treatment of Cancer and Allied Diseases (Eds: Pack, G.T. and Ariel, I.M.) Harper and Row, New York, Vol. 4:591-599, 1960.

111. Wilson, S.E. Esophagogastrectomy Versus Radiation Therapy for Midesophageal Carcinoma. Ann Thorac Surg 10:195-202, 1970.

112. Friedman, M., Egan, J.W. and Southard, M.E. High-Energy Radiation Treatment of Esophageal Cancer. Treatment of Cancer and Allied Diseases (Eds: Pack, G.T. and Ariel, I.M.) Harper and Row, New York, Vol. 4:611-620, 1960.

113. Pearson, J.G. The Radiotherapy of Carcinoma of the Oesophagus and Postcricoid Region in Southeast Scotland. Clin Radiol 17:242-257, 1966.

114. Pearson, J.G. The Value of Radiotherapy in the Management of Esophageal Cancer. Am J Roentgenol 105:500-513, 1969.

115. Pearson, J. G. The Value of Radiotherapy in the Management of Squamous Oesophageal Cancer. Br J Surg 58:794-798, 1971.

116. Pearson, J. G. The Present Status and Future Potential of Radiotherapy in the Management of Esophageal Cancer. Cancer 39:882-890, 1977.

117. McCormack, R. J. M., Edinburgh: Personal Communications.

118. Rider, W. D., Mendoza, R. and Diaz, J. Some Opinions on Treatment of Cancer of the Esophagus. Am J Roentgenol 105:514-517, 1969.

119. Watson, T. A. Radiation Treatment of Cancer of the Esophagus. Surg Gynecol Obstet 117:346-354, 1963.

120. Millburn, L., Faber, L. P. and Hendrickson, F. R. Curative Treatment of Epidermoid Carcinoma of the Esophagus. Am J Roentgen 103:291-299, 1968.

121. Humphrey, C. R. and Cliffton, E. E. Carcinoma of the Distal Part of the Esophagus and Cardia of the Stomach. Surg Gynecol Obstet 128:737-743, 1968.

122. Muggia, F. M. and Cassileth, P. A. Constrictive Pericarditis Following Radiation Therapy. Am J Med 44:116-123, 1968.

123. Nakayama, K., Orihata, H. and Yamaguchi, K. Surgical Treatment Combined with Preoperative Concentrated Irradiation for Esophageal Cancer. Cancer 20:778-788, 1967.

124. Nakayama, K. and Kinoshita, Y. Surgical Treatment Combined with Preoperative Concentrated Radiation: Cancer of the Gastrointestinal Tract. II. Esophagus: Treatment - Localized and Advanced. JAMA 227:178-181, 1974.

125. Akakura, I., Nakamura, Y., Kakegawa, T., Nakayama, R., Watanabe, H. and Yamashita, H. Surgery of Carcinoma of the Esophagus with Preoperative Radiation. Chest 57:47-57, 1970.

126. Parker, E. F. and Gregorie, H. B., Jr. Combined Radiation and Surgical Treatment of Carcinoma of the Esophagus. Ann Surg 161:710-722, 1965.

127. Parker, E. F., Gregorie, H. B., Jr., Arrants, J. E. and Ranvenel, J. M. Carcinoma of the Esophagus. Ann Surg 171:746-751, 1970.

128. Parker, E. F., Gregorie, H. B., Jr. Carcinoma of the Esophagus. Long Term Results. JAMA 235:1018-1020, 1976.

129. Groves, L. K. and Rodriguez-Antunez, A. Treatment of Carcinoma of the Esophagus and Gastric Cardia with Concentrated Preoperative Irradiation Followed by Early Operation: A Progress Report. Ann Thorac Surg 15:333-338, 1973.

130. Fraser, R. W., Wara, W. M., Thomas, A. N., Mauch, P. M., Fishman, N. H., Galante, M., Phillips, T. L. and Buschke, F. Combined Treatment Methods for Carcinoma of the Esophagus. Radiology 128:461-465, 1978.

131. Kasai, M., Mori, S., and Watanabe, T. Follow-up Results After Resection of Thoracic Esophageal Carcinoma. World J Surg 2:543-551, 1978.

132. Dickison, J. C. Palliative Gastrostomy for Inoperable Car-Cinoma of the Esophagus. Can Med Assoc J 65:35-36, 1951.

133. King, T. C. and Zimmerman, J. M. Gastrostomies in Patients with Incurable Cancer. Am Surg 31:251-253, 1965.

134. Heit, H. A., Johnson, L. F., Siegel, S. R. and Boyce, H. W., Jr. Palliative Dilatation for Dysphagia in Esophageal Carcinoma. Ann Intern Med 89:629-631, 1978.

135. Celestin, L. R. Permanent Intubation in Inoperable Cancer of the Oesophagus and Cardia. Ann R Coll Surg Engl 25: 165-169, 1959.

136. Gallagher, E. G., Zumbro, G. L. and Treasure, R. L. Celestin Tube Intubation for Advanced Esophageal Carcinoma. Am J Surg 136:405-407, 1978.

137. Holden, M. P., Wooler, G. H. and Ionescu, M. I. Mousseau-Barbin Tubes for the Treatment of Carcinoma of the Lower Two-Thirds of the Oesophagus: Results and Operative Techniques. Br J Surg 60:401-402, 1973.

138. Thomas, A. N. Treatment of Malignant Esophageal Obstruction by Endoesophageal Intubation. Am J Surg 128:306-314, 1974.

139. Saunders, N. R. The Celestin Tube in the Palliation of Carcinoma of the Esophagus and Cardia. Br J Surg 66:419-421, 1979.

140. Rao, D. D. Celestin Intubation of the Oesophagus. J R Coll Surg Edinb 23:98-99, 1978.

141. Atkinson, M. and Ferguson, R. Fiberoptic Endoscopic Palliative Intubation of Inoperable Oesophagogastric Neoplasms. Br Med J 1:266-267, 1977.

142. Palmer, E. D. Peroral Prosthesis for the Management of Incurable Esophageal Carcinoma. Am J Gastroenterol 59: 487-498, 1973.

143. Hegarty, M. M., Angorn, I. B., Bryer, J. V., Henderson, B. J., LeRoux, B. T., and Logan, A. Pulsion Intubation for Palliation of Carcinoma of the Oesophagus. Br J Surg 64: 160-165, 1977.

144. Lolley, D. M., Jefferson, F. R., Ransdell, H. T., Razzuk, M. A. and Urschel, H. C., Jr. Management of Malignant Esophagorespiratory Fistula. Ann Thorac Surg 25:516-520, 1978.

145. Hegarty, M. M., Angorn, I. B., Bryer, J. V., Henderson, B. J., LeRoux, B. T. and Logan, A. Palliation of Malignant Esophagorespiratory Fistulae by Permanent Indwelling Prosthetic Tube. Ann Surg 185:88-91, 1977.

146. Angorn, I. B., Hegarty, M. M. and Baker, L. W. Palliative Intubation and Resection in Oesophageal Carcinoma. J R Coll Surg Edinb 22:325-330, 1977.

147. Hankins, J. R., Cole, F. N., Attar, S. and McLaughlin, J. S. Carcinoma of the Esophagus: Experience with a Philosophy for Palliation. Ann Thorac Surg 23:400-408, 1977.

148. Ong, G. B. The Kirschner Operation: A Forgotten Procedure. Br J Surg 60:221-227, 1973.

149. Goldsmith, H. S., and Akiyama, H. A Comparative Study of Japanese and American Gastric Dimensions. Ann Surg 190: 690-693, 1979.

150. Orringer, M. B. and Sloan, H. Substernal Gastric Bypass of the Excluded Thoracic Esophagus for Palliation of Esophageal Carcinoma. J Thorac Cardiovasc Surg 70:836-851, 1975.

151. Akiyama, H., Miyazono, H., Tsurumaru, M., Hashimoto, C. and Kawamura, T. Use of the Stomach as an Esophageal Substitute. Ann Surg 188:606-610, 1978.

152. Wilkins, E. W. and Burke, J. F. Colon Esophageal Bypass. Am J Surg 129:394-400, 1975.

153. Nichols, R. E., Broido, P., Condon, R. E., Gorbach, S. L. and Nyhus, L. M. Effect of Preoperative Neomycin-Erythromycin Intestinal Preparation on the Incidence of Infectious Complications Following Colon Surgery. Ann Surg 178:453-458, 1973.

154. Mullen, D. C., Postlethwait, R. W. and Dillon, M. L. Complications of Substernal Colon Interposition. Am Surg 36:80-84, 1970.

155. Belsey, R. Reconstruction of the Esophagus with Left Colon. J Thorac Cardiovasc Surg 49:33-53, 1965.

156. Petrov, B. A. Retrosternal Artificial Esophagus Created from Colon. Surgery 55:520-523, 1964.

157. Comis, R. L. and Carter, S. K. A Review of Chemotherapy in Gastric Cancer. Cancer 34:1576-1586, 1974.

158. Moertel, C. G., O'Connell, M. J. and Lavin, P. T. Chemotherapy of Gastric Carcinoma. Proc Am Assoc Cancer Res 20:288, 1979.

159. MacDonald, J. S., Schein, P. S., Woolley, P. V., Goiron, M., Gisselbrecht, C., Brunet, R. and Lagarde, C. 5-Fluorouracil, Mitomycin-C and Adriamycin (FAM) Combination Chemotherapy Results in 61 Patients with Advanced Gastric Cancer. Proc Am Soc Clin Oncol 20:396, 1979.

160. Legha, S. S., Muggia, F. M. and Carter, S. K. Adjuvant Chemotherapy in Lung Cancer. Cancer 39:1415-1424, 1977.

161. Chahinian, A. P., Mandel, E. M., Jaffrey, I. S., Ratner, L. H., Teirstein, A. S. and Holland, J. F. Chemotherapy with or without Immunotherapy in Bronchogenic Carcinoma. Proc Am Soc Clin Oncol 18:333, 1977.

162. Bitran, J. D., Desser, R. K., DeMeester, T. R., Colman, M., Evans, R., Billings, A., Griem, M., Rubenstein, L., Shapiro, C. and Golomb, H. M. Cyclophosphamide, Adriamycin, Methotrexate and Procarbazine (CAMP)-Effective Four-Drug Combination Chemotherapy for Metastatic Non-Oat Cell Bronchogenic Carcinoma. Cancer Treat Rep 60: 1225-1230, 1976.

163. Carter, S. K. The Chemotherapy of Head and Neck Cancer. Semin Oncol 4:413-424, 1977.

164. Wittes, R. E., Cvitkovic, E., Shah, J., Gerold, F. and Strong, E. W. Cisdiamminedichloroplatinum (II)(DDP) in the Treatment of Epidermoid Carcinoma of the Head and Neck. Cancer Treat Rep 61:359-366, 1977.

165. Randolph, V. L., Vallejo, A., Spiro, R. H., Shah, J., Strong, E. W., Huvos, A. G. and Wittes, R. E. Combination Therapy of Advanced Head and Neck Cancer. Cancer 41:460-467, 1978.

166. Kaplan, B. H., Vogl, S. E., Chiuten, D., Lanham, R. and Wollner, D. Chemotherapy of Advanced Cancer of the Head and Neck with Methotrexate, Bleomycin and Cis-Diamminedichloroplatinum in Combination. Proc Am Soc Clin Oncol 20:384, 1979.

167. Elias, E. G., Chretien, P. B., Monnard, E., Khan, T., Bouchelle, W. H., Wiernik, P. H., Lipson, S. D., Hande, K. R. and Zentai, T. Chemotherapy Prior to Local Therapy in Advanced Squamous Cell Carcinoma of the Head and Neck. Cancer 43:1025-1031, 1979.

168. Takita, H., Marabella, P. C., Edgerton, F. and Rizzo, D. Cis-Dichlorodiammineplatinum (II), Adriamycin, Cyclophosphamide, CCNU and Vincristine in Nonsmall Cell Lung Carcinoma: A Preliminary Report. Cancer Treat Rep 63:29-33, 1979.

169. Holter, A. R. and Fischer, J. E. The Effects of Perioperative Hyperalimentation on Complications in Patients with Carcinoma and Weight Loss. J Surg Res 23:31-34, 1977.

170. Conti, S., West, J. P., Fitzpatrick, H. F. Mortality and Morbidity After Esophagogastrectomy for Cancer of the Esophagus and Cardia. Am Surg 43:92-96, 1977.

171. Moghissi, K., Hornshaw, J., Teasdale, P.R. and Dawes, E.A. Parenteral Nutrition in Carcinoma of the Esophagus Treated by Surgery: Nitrogen Balance and Clinical Studies. Brit J Surg 64:125-128, 1977.

172. Haffejee, A.A. and Angorn, I.B. Nutritional Status and the Nonspecific Cellular and Humoral Immune Response in Esophageal Carcinoma. Ann Surg 189:475-479, 1979.

173. Hoover, H.C., Ryan, J.A., Anderson, E.J. and Fischer, J.E. Nutritional Benefits of Immediate Postoperative Jejunal Feeding of an Elemental Diet. Am J Surg 139:153-159, 1980.

174. Andros, G. Blood-Volume and Weight-Loss in Malignant Oesophageal Obstruction. Br J Surg 56:91-95, 1969.

175. Adams, W.E. The Surgical Treatment of Carcinoma of the Esophagus: Need for a More Aggressive Attitude. J Thorac Cardiovasc Surg 50:141-144, 1965.

176. Johnson, C.L. and Clagett, O.T. Palliative Esophagogastrostomy for Inoperable Carcinoma of the Esophagogastric Junction. J Thorac Cardiovasc Surg 60:269-274, 1970.

177. Logan, A. The Surgical Treatment of Carcinoma of the Esophagus and Cardia. J Thorac Cardiovasc Surg 46:150-161, 1963.

178. Carey, J.S., Plested, W.G. and Hughes, R.K. Esophagogastrectomy: Superiority of the Combined Abdominal-Right Thoracic Approach (Lewis Operation). Ann Thorac Surg 14:59-68, 1972.

179. Fischer, R.D., Brawley, R.K. and Kieffer, R.F. Esophagogastrectomy in the Treatment of the Distal Two-Thirds of the Esophagus: Clinical Experience and Operative Methods. Ann Thorac Surg 14:658-670, 1972.

180. Lewis, I. The Surgical Treatment of Carcinoma of the Oesophagus: With Special Reference to a New Operation for Growths of the Middle Third. Br J Surg 34:18-31, 1946.

181. Churchill, E.D. and Sweet, R.H. Transthoracic Resection of Tumors of the Stomach and Esophagus. Ann Surg 115:897-920, 1942.

182. Garlock, J. H. and Klein, S. H. The Surgical Treatment of Carcinoma of the Esophagus and Cardia: An Analysis of 457 Cases. Ann Surg 139:19-34, 1951.

183. Angorn, I. B. Oesophagogastrostomy without a Drainage Procedure in Oesophageal Carcinoma. Br J Surg 62:601-604, 1975.

184. Smith, R. A. Transthoracic Extended Total Gastrectomy for Malignant Obstruction of the Cardio-Oesophageal Junction. Br J Surg 61:524-532, 1974.

185. Petrovsky, B. V. and Vantsian, E. N. Our Experience in the Surgical Treatment of Malignant and Benign Esophageal Tumors. Surgery 62:833-838, 1967.

186. Collis, J. L. The Long-Term Clinical State After Resection with Gastroesophagostomy. Surgery of the Oesophagus: The Coventry Conference. (Eds: Smith, R. A., Smith, R. E.) Butterworths, London, pp. 19-21, 1972.

187. Kock, N. G., Lewin, E. and Petterson, S. Partial or Total Gastrectomy for Adenocarcinoma of the Cardia. Acta Chir Scand 135:340-344, 1969.

188. Hawley, P. R., Westerholm, P. and Morson, B. C. Pathology and Prognosis of Carcinoma of the Stomach. Br J Surg 57:877-883, 1970.

189. Parker, E. F., Ballinger, J. F. and Shull, K. C. Esophageal Resection and Replacement for Carcinoma. Ann Surg 187: 629-633, 1978.

190. Inberg, M. V. and Scheinin, T. M. The Surgery of Esophageal and High Gastric Carcinoma. Ann Chir Gynaecol Fenn 58:197-203, 1969.

191. McCormack, R. J. M. and Walbaum, P. R. Edinburgh: Personal Communications.

192. Postlethwait, R. W., Weinberg, M., Jenkins, L. B. and Brockington, W. S. Mechanical Strength of Esophageal Anastomosis. Ann Surg 133:472-480, 1951.

193. Nance, F. C. New Techniques of Gastrointestinal Anastomoses with the EEA Stapler. Ann Surg 189:587-598, 1979.

194. Steichen, F. M. and Ravitch, M. M. Mechanical Sutures in Esophageal Surgery. Ann Surg 191:373-381, 1980.

195. Bombeck, C. T., Coelho, R. G. P. and Nyhus, L. M. Prevention of Gastroesophageal Reflux After Resection of the Lower Esophagus. Surg Gynecol Obstet 130:1035-1043, 1970.

196. Butterfield, W. C. Anti-Reflux Palliative Resections for Inoperable Carcinoma of the Esophagogastric Junction. J Thorac Cardiovasc Surg 62:460-464, 1971.

197. Butterfield, W. C. Gastric Fundoplication in Esophageal Surgery Other Than Hiatal Hernia Repairs: A Review of Experimental Studies and Clinical Applications. Rev Surg 30: 77-83, 1972.

198. Boyd, A. D., Cukingnan, R., Engleman, R. M., Localio, S. A., Slattery, L., Tice, D. A., Bardin, J. A. and Spencer, F. C. Esophagogastrostomy: Analysis of 55 Cases. J Thorac Cardiovasc Surg 70:817-825, 1975.

199. Allison, P. R. and da Silva, L. T. The Roux Loop. Br J Surg 41:173-180, 1953.

200. Efskind, L. and Helsingen, N. Carcinoma of the Lower Portion of the Esophagus. Acta Chir Scand (Suppl) 356:110-120, 1965.

201. Zacho, A. and Fischermann, K. Surgical Treatment of Malignancies of the Oesophagogastric Junction. Acta Chir Scand (Suppl) 356:121-129, 1965.

202. Magill, T. G. and Simmons, R. L. Resection of Cardioesophageal Carcinoma: Factors Contributing to its Mortality, Palliation, and Cure. Arch Surg 94:865-870, 1967.

203. Appelqvist, P., Mattila, S., Jyrala, A. and Tala, P. Surgical Treatment of Carcinoma of the Oesophagus and Cardia. Scand J Thorac Cardiovasc Surg 11:278-282, 1977.

204. Jackson, J. W., Cooper, D. K. C., Guvendik, L. and Reece-Smith, H. The Surgical Management of Malignant Tumours of the Oesophagus and Cardia: A Review of the Results in 292 Patients Treated Over a 15 Year Period (1961-1975). Br J Surg 66:98-104, 1979.

205. Maillard, J. N., Launois, B., deLagausie, Ph., Lellouch, J., Lortat-Jacob, J. L. Cause of Leakage at the Site of Anastomosis After Esophagogastric Resection for Carcinoma. Surg Gynecol Obstet 129:1014-1018, 1969.

206. Steiger, Z., Nichel, W. O., Wilson, R. F. and Arbulu, A. Improved Surgical Palliation of Advanced Carcinoma of the Esophagus. Am J Surg 135:782-784, 1978.

207. Piccone, V. A., LeVeen, H. H., Ahmed, N. and Grosberg, S. Reappraisal of Esophagogastrectomy for Esophageal Malignancy. Am J Surg 137:32-38, 1979.

208. Sweet, R. H. The Results of Treatment of Carcinoma of the Esophagus. JAMA 155:422-431, 1954.

209. Dietrich, R. A., Dockerty, M. B., Olsen, A. M. and Ellis, F. H., Jr. Clinicopathologic Study of Carcinoma Involving the Esophagogastric Junction. Surg Gynecol Obstet 118: 1223-1233, 1964.

210. Collis, L. H. Surgical Treatment of Carcinoma of the Oesophagus and Cardia. Br J Surg 58:801-804, 1971.

211. Borst, H. G., Dragojevic, D., Stegmann, T. and Hetzer, R. Anastomotic Leakage, Stenosis, and Reflux After Esophageal Replacement. World J Surg 2:861-866, 1978.

212. Payne, W. S. The Long-Term Clinical State After Resection with Total Gastrectomy and Roux Loop Anastomosis. Surgery of the Esophagus: The Coventry Conference. (Eds: Smith, R. A. and Smith, R. E.) Butterworths, London, pp. 23-28, 1972.

213. Gunning, A. J. The Long-Term Clinical State After Resection with Jejunal Replacement. Surgery of the Esophagus: The Coventry Conference. (Eds: Smith, R. A. and Smith, R. E.) Butterworths, London, pp. 29-33, 1972.

214. Johnson, L. F. and DeMeester, T. R. Twenty-four Hour pH Monitoring of the Distal Esophagus: A Quantitative Measure of Gastroesophageal Reflux. Am J Gastroenterol 62:325-331, 1974.

215. Lam, K. H., Lim, S. T. K., Wong, J., Lam, S. K. and Ong, G. B. Gastric Histology and Function in Patients with Intrathoracic Stomach Replacement After Esophagectomy. Surgery 85:283-290, 1979.

216. Ward, A. S. and Collis, J. L. Late Results of Oesophageal and Oesophagogastric Resection in the Treatment of Oesophageal Cancer. Thorax 26:1-5, 1971.

217. Inberg, M. V., Markkanen, T., Scheinin, T. M. and Harri, J. Absorption Studies After Excisional Surgery of Esophageal and High Gastric Carcinoma. Acta Chir Scand 136:509-516, 1970.

INDEX

Achalasia, 5, 18, 28
Adenocarcinoma, 1, 13, 87-88, 106, 108
Age of the patient:
  epidemiological factor, 3
  risk factor for surgery, 43-44
Alcohol, see Epidemiology
Anastomosis, esophagogastric, see Esophagogastric anastomosis
Anastomotic leakage, 65-66, 104-105, 107, 109
Anastomotic stricture, 109-110
Anemia, 4, 16, 112-113
  iron deficiency, 16, 112-113
  pernicious, 4, 112-113
Arterial blood gases, 17, 44, 102
Atrophic gastritis, 5, 111

Barium esophagogram, 17-18, 21-37, 40
  configurations:
    infiltrative, 17-18, 22, 31
    polyploid, 18, 23
    ulcerative, 18
  corner sign, 18, 25-26
  differential diagnosis, 18, 28
  esophageal axis, 40-41
Bleeding as a symptom, 9, 15
Blood group A, see Epidemiology
Bone metastases, see Metastases
Bone scan, 18-19

Cartilage incision, 80-81, 101, 111
Caustic stricture:
  differential diagnosis, 18, 33
  epidemiological factor, 5
Celestin tube, 55-57, 59-60
  technique of insertion, 55-57
Chemotherapy, 67-68
Chronic obstructive pulmonary disease, see Pulmonary disease
Colon interposition, 61-66, 71, 77, 88, 100, 110
  complications of, 65-66
  preparation for, 71
  results of, 65-66, 110
  technique of, 62-66
Computerized axial tomography scan (CAT scan), 42
Cough as a symptom, 9, 15

Decreasing frequency of gastroesophageal carcinoma, 3
Definition of gastroesophageal carcinoma, 1
Dehydration, 69-71
Diaphragm incision, 80, 82, 101
Diet as an epidemiological factor, 3-7
Dilatation of gastroesophageal cancer, 54, 110
Distant metastases, see Metastases
Dumping syndrome, 111-112
Dysphagia, 8, 14-15, 43, 48, 54-68, 74-78, 110
  palliation of, 43, 54-68, 74-78, 110
  as a symptom, 8, 14-15

EEA stapler use in esophagogastrostomy, 93-94
Epidemiology of gastroesophageal carcinoma, 2-7
  age, 3
  decreasing frequency, 3
  geographic variation, 2-3, 6
  mineral deficiencies, 4, 6
  nitrosamines and nitrosamides, 5-7
  race variations, 3
  risk factors:
    achalasia, 5
    alcohol, 3-4, 6, 8
    atrophic gastritis, 5
    blood group A, 4
    caustic strictures, 5
    diet, 3-7
    low socioeconomic class, 3-4
    pernicious anemia, 4
    previous gastric surgery, 4-5
    reflux esophagitis, 4
    tobacco, 3-4, 6
  sex variations, 3
  vitamin deficiencies, 4, 6
Esophageal biopsy, 18-19
Esophageal layers, 90-91
Esophagitis, see Reflux esophagitis
Esophagogastric anastomosis, 90-96
Esophagogastrostomy, 77-78, 88-96
  technique of, 89-96
Esophagojejunostomy (Roux loop), 77-78, 88, 96-100
  technique of, 96-100
Esophagorespiratory fistula (Tracheo-

esophageal fistula), 16, 59-60, 77
Esophagoscopy, 18-19, 38, 39-40

Fundoplication, 95-97, 109-110

Gastrectomy, partial versus total, 88
Gastroesophageal anastomosis, see Esophagogastric anastomosis
Gastrostomy, 54, 70
Geographic distribution of gastroesophageal carcinoma, 2-3, 6

Heart disease as a risk factor, 45-46, 101-102, 104-106
Histology of gastroesophageal carcinoma:
adenocarcinoma, 1, 13, 87-88, 106, 108
carcinosarcoma, 2
lymphosarcoma, 2
oat cell carcinoma, 2
rhabdomyosarcoma, 2
squamous carcinoma, 1, 13, 87-88, 106, 108
Hyperalimentation, see Intravenous hyperalimentation
Hypercalcemia, 10-11

Incidence of gastroesophageal carcinoma, see Epidemiology
"Inkwell" anastomosis, 95
Inoperable, 8, 11, 69
Intravenous hyperalimentation, 70, 103
Intubation, see Prosthetic intubation

Jejunostomy, 70

Laboratory studies, 16-17, 42
Laparotomy, 42-43, 72-78
Leakage, anastomotic, see Anastomotic leakage
Liver function tests, 17-19, 42
Liver metastases, see Metastases
Liver scan, 18-19, 42
Local spread, see Metastases
Lung metastases, see Metastases
Lymphatic metastases, see Metastases

Malnutrition, see Weight loss
Mediastinoscopy, 40, 42, 69
Metastases:
adrenal, 10, 106-109
bone, 10, 18-19, 106-109
distant (blood borne), 10-11, 16, 40-43, 73-78, 106-109
liver, 10, 16-19, 42-43, 73-80
local spread, 9, 11, 40-43, 73-80, 88, 106-109
submucosal, 9, 88
lung, 10, 17, 69, 106-109
lymphatic, 10, 15-16, 40-43, 69, 73-80, 106-109
tracheal or bronchial, 16, 59-60, 69
Mineral deficiencies, 4, 6
Monitoring, 72, 102
Mousseau-Barbin tube, 55

Natural history of gastroesophageal carcinoma, 8-13
Nitrosamines and nitrosamides, 5-7

Pain as a symptom, 9, 15
Palliation, 12, 43, 54-68, 69, 75-77
bypass procedure, 61-66
colon interposition, 61-66
limited esophagogastric bypass (Johnson-Claggett), 76-77
subcutaneous stomach tube (Kirschner), 61
substernal stomach bypass, 61
dilatation, 55-56
of esophagorespiratory fistula, 59-60
gastrostomy, 54
intubation, 56-60, 75-77
pulsion tube, 57-60, 69, 75
technique of insertion, 57-59
traction tube, 55-57, 59-60, 75-77
technique of insertion, 55-57
radiation, 60-61, 69, 75-77, 110
surgical resection, 61
Palmer tube, 55
Post thoracotomy pain, 111
Proctor-Livingstone tube, 55, 57-60, 69, 110
technique of insertion, 57-59
Prosthetic intubation of gastroesophageal carcinoma, 56-60
of esophagorespiratory fistula, 59-60
pulsion tube, 57-60, 69, 110
traction tube, 55-57, 59-60
Pulmonary disease, 17, 44-45
Pulmonary function tests, 17, 44-45
Pulmonary hygiene, 71, 101-102

Race variations, see Epidemiology
Radiation therapy:
combined with surgery:
preoperative, 49-50
postoperative, 51, 110
palliative, 60-61, 69, 75-77, 110
radical (curative), 47-49, 51, 76-77

Radiological diagnosis, see Barium esophagogram
Reflux esophagitis:
  epidemiological factor, 4
  postoperative, 109-110
Resection margins, 10, 88
Risk factors:
  in etiology of gastroesophageal carcinoma, see Epidemiology
  for surgical resection, 43-46
    age, 43-44
    cirrhosis, 46
    heart disease, 45-46
    peripheral vascular disease, 46
    previous surgical procedures, 46-47
    pulmonary disease, 44-45
Roux loop (Roux-en-Y esophagojejunostomy), see Esophagojejunostomy

Scleroderma, 5, 18, 32
Selective therapy, 39-68
Selective therapy scheme, 52-53, 68
Signs of gastroesophageal carcinoma, 15-16
Souttar tube, 55
Squamous carcinoma, 1, 13, 87-88, 106, 108
Staging of gastroesophageal carcinoma, 11-13, 39-43, 72-78
  laparotomy for, 42-43, 72-78
  TMN system of, 11-13
Stomach for esophageal replacement:
  esophagogastrectomy, 77-78, 88-96
  limited esophagogastric bypass (Johnson-Claggett), 76-77
  subcutaneous stomach tube (Kirschner), 61
  substernal stomach tube, 61
Stricture, anastomotic, see Anastomotic stricture
Surgical resection of gastroesophageal carcinoma:
  complications of, 103-113
    early, 104-106
    late, 106-113
  contraindications to (inoperable), 8, 11, 69
  inability to resect (unresectable), 12, 74-77, 79
  incision for, 78-80, 100-101
  mortality of, 104-109
  palliative resection, 12, 61
  preoperative preparations for, 69-72
  postoperative care, 101-103
  pyloric division, 89
  radical resection (curative), 12, 51, 78-101
    technique of, 78-101
  results of, 103-113
Surgical resection and radiation therapy, see Radiation therapy
Survival statistics, 12, 47-51, 104-109
Symptoms of gastroesophageal carcinoma, 14-15

Tobacco, see Epidemiology
Tracheoesophageal fistula, see Esophagorespiratory fistula

Unresectable, 12, 74-77, 79-80

Vitamin deficiencies, see Epidemiology

Weight loss as a symptom, 15, 69-71